THE

YOGA
BODY
DIET

THE

YOGA

BODY

DIET

SLIM AND SEXY IN 4 WEEKS

(WITHOUT THE STRESS)

KRISTEN SCHULTZ DOLLARD

AND JOHN DOUILLARD, DC, PHD

WITH JENNIFER ISERLOH

RODALE

This book is intended as a reference volume only, not as a medical manual. The information given here is designed to help you make informed decisions about your health. It is not intended as a substitute for any treatment that may have been prescribed by your doctor. If you suspect that you have a medical problem, we urge you to seek competent medical help. The information in this book is meant to supplement, not replace, proper exercise training. All forms of exercise pose some inherent risks. The editors and publisher advise readers to take full responsibility for their safety and know their limits. Before practicing the exercises in this book, be sure that your equipment is well-maintained, and do not take risks beyond your level of experience, aptitude, training, and fitness. The exercise and dietary programs in this book are not intended as a substitute for any exercise routine or dietary regimen that may have been prescribed by your doctor. As with all exercise and dietary programs, you should get your doctor's approval before beginning.
Mention of specific companies, organizations, or authorities in this book does not imply endorsement by the author or publisher, nor does mention of specific companies, organizations, or authorities imply that they endorse this book, its author, or the publisher.
Internet addresses and telephone numbers given in this book were accurate at the time it went to press.

Library of Congress Cataloging-in-Publication Data

Dollard, Kristen Schultz.
    The yoga body diet : slim and sexy in 4 weeks (without the stress) / Kristen Schultz Dollard and John Douillard ; with Jennifer Iserloh.
        p.   cm.
    Includes index.
    ISBN-13 978–1–60529–648–7 pbk.
    1. Hatha yoga.   2. Health.   3. Nutrition.   4. Exercise.   I. Douillard, John.   II. Iserloh, Jennifer.   III. Title.
RA781.7D65   2010
613.7′046—dc22
                            2010004948

Distributed to the trade by Macmillan

2 4 6 8 10 9 7 5 3 1   paperback

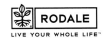

We inspire and enable people to improve their lives and the world around them

For more of our products visit **rodalestore.com** or call 800-848-4735

For Avery, my little life force;

and Terry, for sending me to a yoga school all those years ago;

and Mom, for everything.

—Kristen Dollard

Whether contemplating your first yoga class or a master of the mat;
whether frustrated with your weight or just way too stressed, *The Yoga Body Diet* is dedicated to
your journey—one aimed at perfect health and the joy of living.

—John Douillard

CONTENTS

ACKNOWLEDGEMENTS

First and foremost, to all of those people who touched this project, who were willing to look at yoga and reinvent it's image to be both mainstream and simple without sacrificing a pound of its power to improve your body, mind, and heart.

I am most grateful to the team whose expertise created a brain trust for this book. Thank you to my editor Shannon Welch for championing the project and for your tenacity around translating yoga for a mainstream audience. Paige Greenfield, your biblical consistency and writing chops invigorated the experience. Jennifer Iserloh, without your boundless commitment to and fluency with fresh, healthy delicious food, the menu would be mung bean stew 75 ways. And John Douillard, you are more healer than doctor and more human than any doctor I've ever known. To all the women who test drove the diet, this book is for you.

I am infinitely grateful to Rodale and the Rodale family for being the kind of place where yoga is as much a part of the culture as newsstand sales. Steve Murphy, thank you for believing in me always and for getting behind the idea that that yoga is as powerful a product as a personal practice. Yes, you have yoga cred.

A special thanks to everyone—and there were many—who made *YogaLife* magazine and iyogalife.com the platform from which this book came. Not the least of whom is Bill Stump, who championed yoga at Rodale (and does yoga in his basement.) Bill thanks for supporting me and your editorial heroics. And to those who made my yoga life one of the best professional experiences I'll ever have not to mention a site with yoga cred: Nicole Kwan, John Capouya, Siobhan Hardy Royer, Jessica Levine, Dana Meltzer Zepeda, Sean Nolan, and Brunello Creative.

I wanted to thank those people who have supported me in my career because in leading by example you've been the kind of people I didn't think existed in corporate America. Your high standards, smarts, and commitment to showing up have kept me in the game. "Cosmic" Robin Ormsby, Ann Pleshette Murphy, Bill Stump, David Willey, Steve Madden, and Michelle Meyercord thank you.

To my yoga teachers Baron Baptiste, Seane Corn, Jean Koerner, and Mary Wirick I offer a humble thank you. I am in your debt. You have inspired me to be and do more on and off the mat. Anything I say here would be inadequate so simply, "Namaste."

To Nancy Lonsdorf who was my first Ayurvedic doctor when some physicians questioned my fertility. Your wise water is powerful stuff. I believe Avery is here, in part, because of your recipe for health.

For my friends and family, you know who you are. Mom, Dad, Bill, John, and Pete—I love you guys. Thanks for loving me back and supporting me. This book helped me realize that I have the kind of family some people only dream of having. Mom, thanks for artfully setting the Schultz family health standards so high without making us feel no-sugar cereal was anything but normal. Your teachings have served our families and us so well.

I would be incomplete if I did not thank the friends who supported me as I struggled to balance writing a book, motherhood, wifedom, and a full time job—not to mention some yoga teaching on the side. Jenny Dee (and Uncle Paul), Laura, Fama, "My Chicas," and the Koffs and the Thomisons (our commune). And Erica, because I know you're always out there and I love you. And a special thanks to Nila and Kirit Shah and "Ba." Thanks for bringing India to me. It was at your house the tastes, smells and symbols of India connected me to yoga's birthplace. What a gift.

And to all of my yoga students: especially Lina, Johanna, Steve, and Jane, your energy is sustaining. Thanks for letting me and yoga into your life.

Terry and Avery, thanks for the sacrifices you made to help me do this. How did I get lucky enough to live with two people for whom unconditional love comes so easy?

—*Kristen Dollard*

I would like to thank Kristin Schultz Dollard for inviting me to be a part of this project and whose vision, dedication, and sacrifice became *The Yoga Body Diet*. To my good friend Felicia Tomasko from LA Yoga who referred me to Kristen and the Rodale team. I would like to thank our editor Shannon Welch for being so competent and such a joy to work with. To Paige Greenfield for extracting knowledge out of me that I didn't know I had, and to Jennifer Iserloh whose expertise and recipes have taken this book to a whole other level.

I would like to thank my patients who continually teach me how to speak and listen to the silent language of the human healing system.

And, most important, to my greatest accomplishment: the bond of unconditional love I enjoy with my incredible wife and teacher Ginger and our six children, Janaki, Devaki, Austin, Mason, Jensen, and Gigi.

—*John Douillard*

Your Guide to Building a Yoga Body

(It's Not as Hard as You Think.)

The first fruits of the practice of yoga are health,
little waste matter, and a clear complexion;
lightness of the body, a pleasant scent, and a sweet voice;
and an absence of greedy desires.
—The Upanishads

A yoga body is the one you have now, only healthier. This book is your complete guide to how to get it. It's not as hard as you might think.

The best part? The benefits don't stop at your appearance. At the end of 4 short weeks, you'll feel better, you'll think more clearly, and you'll find it's much easier to keep a positive mindset and roll with life's inevitable punches. *The Yoga Body Diet* is more than a diet; it's a change in how you relate to yourself and your body. Losing weight is just a fringe benefit—a pretty good one.

These might sound like big promises, but they're grounded in science and rooted in an ancient practice that we've adapted for today's demanding lifestyles.

A Brief History of Yoga

Although the first book on yoga, *The Yoga Sutras*, was published 2,000 years ago, it is estimated that people have been practicing yoga for 5,000 years. Yoga comes from the Sanskrit word *yuj*, meaning "yoke" or "union," describing the connection—the union—between body, mind, and spirit. A typical yoga class includes physical postures (called *asanas*), breath control exercises (called *pranayamas*), and sometimes meditation and philosophy.

The pretzel-tying, incense-burning, and spiritually proselytizing aspects of yoga get a lot of press, but the truth is that in America today, 25 million people say they will try yoga in the next year. And the reason is this: It is a perfect way to de-stress. Last year, millions of Americans—some 13 million, in fact—took a yoga class and discovered that it isn't too hard, and it isn't scary. What else they did they report? It's a good workout, it feels fantastic, and it's better than a massage or martini when it comes to affordable and long-term stress relief.

Thirty-five years ago, Dr. Herbert Benson, Director Emeritus of the Benson-Henry Institute and Mind/Body Medical Institute at Harvard Medical School, educated America on what he called *the relaxation response*. He administered a battery of tests, measuring blood pressure, brain waves, heart rate, and rate of breathing among practitioners of Transcendental Meditation (the Beatles are the most famous TM practitioners) as they sat quietly for 20 minutes and again while they meditated for 20 minutes. Through the simple act of changing their thought patterns while meditating, the subjects experienced decreases in blood pressure, breathing rate, and heart rate, and had slower brain waves— changes that characterize a relaxation response.

Subsequent studies have revealed that we can tap into this effect through multiple channels. Prayer works. Yoga and deep breathing work. So do running and dicing carrots (although not simultaneously).

Repetition—of a sound, word, or movement— helps to trigger a relaxation response. It also helps to quiet mental chatter. Yoga, a series of movements that are held and repeated in tandem with deep breathing, elicits a relaxation response. One of the main differences between a generic cardio workout and a yoga workout is that if you match your breath to the movement, you'll trigger your relaxation response. That is critical for healing and, in turn, for weight loss. The yoga body diet's bag of tricks sculpts a body and a mindset profoundly different from one that's built in the weight room.

Yoga poses (there are more than 13,000, but our "greatest hits compilation" in Chapter 9 distills the most accessible and user-friendly) use your own body weight and gravity to pull muscle toward the bone, rather than creating muscle tears, which build mass. Yoga creates a body that's more dancer than linebacker. Bulky muscle—the kind most people get by pumping iron—is hungry. It literally requires more calories to keep it from melting into flab. This makes keeping the balance in calorie in–calorie out equation nearly impossible. On the other hand, yoga doesn't leave you famished. After class you do not binge on a buffet of food (or want to, for that matter) and hours later crucify yourself for the caloric inequity. For this reason, this diet is a solution for anyone who exercises like a fiend and still cannot slim down.

Elite physicians, inarguably Western in their approach to medicine, have begun to trumpet yoga's amazing effects. According to the National Institutes of Health, studies have shown yoga to:

- Improve mood
- Counteract stress
- Reduce heart rate and blood pressure
- Increase lung capacity
- Improve muscle relaxation
- Help with conditions such as anxiety, depression, and insomnia
- Improve overall physical fitness, strength, and flexibility
- Positively affect levels of certain brain or blood chemicals

In 2008, researchers in India published a study in the journal *Diabetes Research and Clinical Practice* that found that after 3 months of practicing yoga, participants lost more weight and lowered their blood pressure, triglycerides, and blood sugar levels (all indicators of metabolic speed) more than those who received standard care, such as medication, for their symptoms.

On the mind-body topic, yoga is based on a pretty cool principle called *Ahimsa*, which means

"I'm Not Flexible Enough" and Other Yoga Myths Debunked

We often hear the same refrains when the uninitiated talk about yoga. Here are answers to the most nagging questions.

1. "I'm not flexible."

Yoga is for Gumbys; gyms are for buffies, goes the thinking. In fact, yoga increases flexibility. Many people who thought they'd never be able to touch their toes can do incredible things after just a few deep breaths.

2. "You don't work hard enough in yoga to lose weight."

We now have proof that cutting calories alone doesn't leave you skinny. If you don't change what you eat *and* how you exercise, that scale won't sing. The gym has its place in the world, but it's not all it's cracked up to be (and too time consuming to sustain), and gyms do not actively encourage a ninja-like mind (although being able to zone out in front of seven TVs while treadmilling is masterful, we admit). The mind-body connection is the future of health.

3. "Yoga is a cult of hippies with yuppie money."

We desperately want to show you how yoga is transgenerational, for rich and poor and superficial and profound—just like life. Failing to travel to India, eating meat for protein, or drinking wine doesn't diminish one's ability to understand yoga. Yoga is about increasing your awareness, plunging into your daily life, and turning your future into something so desirable you wake up awash in possibility.

4. "It takes fancy poses to be good at yoga."

The person struggling in the corner is often a lot better at yoga in some ways than the precise, uptight perfectionist in row one. What matters more: mat skills or life skills? Life is lived mostly off the sticky mat, so no matter how awesome your Eagle is, how do you handle Mom's emergency pacemaker surgery happening on the day of your daughter's birthday? Do you have perspective enough to stay productive when the chips are down or you're overwhelmed? Your response to a high-pressure scenario is a better indicator of your yoga than the length of time you hold the Crow pose.

Let go.

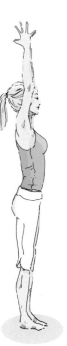

"non-harming" in Sanskrit. The philosophy encourages you to embrace a gentle attitude, and part of this is about being gentle on yourself. You don't have to try to pound your body into shape. In yoga, you respect it, take care of it, and offer it the kind of movement and breathing that it intuitively desires. It's a good place to start going easy on your body. And Ayurveda, yoga's little sister, is built on this exact theory: that the body's intelligence is profound. As a science, Ayurveda is an organic rehab for an imbalanced body.

MEET YOGA'S LITTLE SISTER: AYURVEDA

In one poetic phrase borrowed from a swami, yoga and Ayurveda can be described as "two wings of a dove." While yoga is the exercise science behind building a buff body, its sister science, Ayurveda, plays a starring role in *The Yoga Body Diet*. It is second nature in India. Just like we run out for Emergen-C at a pharmacy, our friends in Bangalore grab trikatu (a digestive powder made with three spices). The Sanskrit word *Ayurveda* translates to "science" (*ayur*) and "life" (*veda*), literally, "the science of life." At 5,000 years old, it is one of the world's oldest medical systems. Today, 80 percent of India's population continues to use Ayurveda exclusively or combined with Western medicine. You've experienced pieces of Ayurveda in disguise. It

was the inspiration for the beauty line Aveda.

The modern applications are many, and some have made headlines, giving Ayurveda a bad rap. One aspect of the plan is herbs, but in *The Yoga Body Diet*, herbs include the pretty greens like mint and tarragon that you can grow on your windowsill. You won't have to ingest a thing by capsule. Our mission is to deliver Ayurveda's greatest hits and to teach you how to use it for weight loss. We've translated and mainstreamed this ancient science. Between the workouts and the recipes and the simplicity of the lifestyle changes, the program will feel as if you hired Hollywood royalty's holistic health counselor to coach you to your new whole-body health goal.

Ayurveda's preventive mission is to purify the mind, body, and soul. Its target: to prevent or remedy digestive problems. According to Ayurveda, diseases often start with improper digestion. When we eat, undigested molecules of food (called *ama*) stick to tissues and, over time, cause damage and destruction. Think about how cholesterol clogs arteries or how cigarette smoke renders lungs black. Ayurveda maintains that if you eat the wrong foods, your body can't be expected to process the impurities, and the result is clogged drains.

You may have experienced this if you have elimination problems, skin rashes or breakouts, irritable bowel syndrome, colitis, or stomach acidity. Why do we suffer from these conditions? According to Ayurveda, it's because the body has been unable to break down ama. As if symptoms of digestive duress weren't hard enough to contend with, the buildup of ama makes it hard for us to burn off bulky fat. The body is too busy to break down fat. Ultimately, if the body is unable to attend to normal processes, illness and disease result.

Ayurveda, in conjunction with a simple yoga practice, detoxifies the body. *The Yoga Body Diet* will cleanse the digestive system and renovate your health. Once the digestive system's plumbing is in working order, the body can get back to breaking down fat, creating energy, and keeping your immunity high.

Ayurveda's main mission is not weight loss. And that's a good thing. Many diet plans may help you achieve weight loss in the short term, but it may come at the expense of the well-being of other bodily systems. You don't want to be thin but on dialysis or skinny but hypoglycemic. Many famous diets have little-known side effects. Stringent weigh-ins and counting calories loosen the grip you have on feeling good. And the harder we try, the harder it becomes to lose weight for good. *The Yoga Body Diet*'s only side effect is mind-body balance.

The impact of Ayurveda and yoga on weight loss is secondary. Ayurveda's real mission is to heal. The underlying philosophy holds that our bodies are intelligent, and that if we pay attention, they will tell us exactly what we need. If eating dairy upsets your stomach, your body is trying to tell you something. If you break out when you eat spicy sauces, your body is trying to send you a sign that something more cooling would be better for your skin.

Given all of the stimulation we're subject to, it's tough to be in tune with our basic needs. Our overtaxed lives have trashed our bodies. How many young guys have colitis now? How many women struggle with infertility? How many of us can't get a good night's sleep?

It's as simple as this: We can't fight fat until we win the war on stress. To do this, we need to listen to our bodies. The best part about yoga and Ayurveda is that they teach us that our intuition and natural inclination can tell us a lot if we slow down enough to put them in the front seat.

This book will help you learn to listen to *your* body and understand that reactions to food and fitness are unique to your individual needs. *The Yoga Body Diet* looks at *how* and *what* to eat as ways to make your body's activities, from digestion to sleep, more effective by restoring whole-body balance in the face of stress. And once your digestion de-stresses, you'll not only have shed unwanted pounds (and your sugar cravings), but your metabolic rate will automatically intensify, and fat won't stand a chance.

GOOD STRESS, BAD STRESS

Why will this plan work where other diets have failed you? *The Yoga Body Diet* identifies stress as a key obstacle to long-term weight loss. And, rather than putting your mind and body under intense duress through extreme and unnatural changes in food and fitness, the program subtracts stress from the get-skinny equation. To cure stress, we have to understand it rather than let it scare us.

Here's the story. Our nervous system has two sides: the sympathetic and parasympathetic. You are familiar with the fight-or-flight response, when stress flips the switch on the sympathetic nervous system. Why might this be good? If you have to race out of a burning building, dodge an oncoming car, or perform a presentation to win your promotion, the sympathetic nervous system controls survival instincts. What happens in your body when survival is at stake is that the pupils dilate, the heart pumps blood fast and furiously, and digestion slows. And because your body translates crisis to mean "no food for long stretches," it stores fat. If you're in the tundra, this is great news. If you're going to be wearing a bridesmaid dress and you're so stressed with work, finances, and relationships that your gym routine isn't shedding the pounds for you, it's not.

The other side of the nervous system, the parasympathetic, is the welcome la-la land of serenity. Stimulating the parasympathetic nervous system has these soothing physiological effects: The heart rate slows, digestion increases, and sexual arousal becomes easier. So our claim on the cover—slim and sexy without stress—is contingent upon how able we are to mellow out our nervous system on command. *The Yoga Body Diet* begins by using yogic techniques to ban cortisol—the bad-for-you chemical produced by stress—using yoga, and teaching you to induce and create reserves of the state of grace we call "calm." How do we do that? By eliciting the relaxation response to soothe the nervous system. If we can begin to bank a little bliss, we can combat stress when it comes calling.

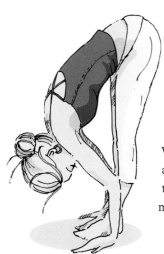

Stress is Fat's Welcome Mat.

We no longer live moments away from death by saber-toothed tigers or woolly mammoths or warring tribes. But our brains still respond to stress as if our lives were on the line, relaying a message to the adrenal glands to secrete a cascade of hormones—among them adrenaline and cortisol. This sends the body into fight-or-flight mode; heart rate and blood pressure skyrocket, enabling you to flee at super-human speeds and to make lifesaving decisions in milliseconds. At the same time, digestion shuts down. After all, when outrunning a predator you probably won't have time to down an energy bar to refuel. In an emergency, you are designed to store fat in case you'll be living off of it.

But here's the catch: Although at times your boss may not seem so different from a prehistoric mammal that sees you as dinner, the war is over. Unfortunately, your body never got the memo. The human body interprets and reacts to stress the same way it has for millions of years, no matter the cause. So, whether it's an overflowing inbox or a loincloth-clad tribe that's stressing you out, the body does the same thing.

Although all of the stress responses exist to save your life, the human body can only sustain so much. Over time, faster heart rate, elevated blood pressure, and increased levels of stress hormones chip away at your immune system and your health. Thus, up to 90 percent of visits to doctors' offices are due to stress-related conditions.

That's what happens to your health, but what about your waistline? Even if you're sweating it out at the gym or monitoring your diet like a nutritionist, the fact remains that if you are stressed out, your body hold onto fat for dear life.

Stress also takes a serious toll on digestion. The digestive system with, among other things, its 22 feet of intestines, isn't the most glamorous aspect of your anatomy. Still, examining how it reacts to stress provides vital information on why even your most valiant weight-loss efforts, if successful, have been fleeting, and why this plan is going to be the last one you'll ever need.

The small intestine contains 7 million *villi*, tiny, finger-like projections that protrude from cells lining the intestinal wall. Their job is to increase the surface area of the intestine in order to facilitate the absorption of nutrients from food as it's being shuttled through your digestive system. Nutrients travel through the villi and get swept up into the bloodstream.

The intestinal wall is also wired with stress receptors. One of the body's many reactions to stress is to form a layer of thick, gooey mucus inside the intestinal wall. (If you've ever experienced an upset stomach when stressed, that's

The Yoga Body Acid Test

A healthy body needs an alkaline environment to flourish. But when stress attacks, it sets off a series of events resulting in a highly acidic state. Losing weight—not to mention maintaining good health—when your body is flooded with acidic chemicals is next to impossible.

Foods with a more basic (in the sense of less acidic) chemistry include vegetables (especially sprouts and leafy greens) and whole grains. This is why you hear about green drinks being the heart and soul of any cleanse. Flushing the body with chards and spinach restores the pH. The right foods can counter the chemical reactions that stress ignites.

Here's a look at how the chemical reactions that stress incites can wreak havoc on your body:

1. Stress signals your adrenal glands (triangular-shaped glands on top of both kidneys) to pump out certain hormones, including cortisol and adrenaline, which are naturally acidic.

2. These chemicals cause you to crave emergency fuel—foods that are dense with fat and calories that would sustain you if you really were being chased by a grizzly. However, since most foods today come off a shelf instead of out of the ground, what we crave is what's most readily available: hamburgers, cheese fries, sundaes, and margaritas. On top of that, we're hardwired to crave them. In a study where researchers subjected rats to chronic stress and then offered them nutrition-rich chow or a mixture of sugar and fat, they chose the latter every time. One thing all comfort foods have in common (besides being delicious): They are acidic and shift your body's pH.

3. Why is your body unable to shed weight in an acidic environment? First, the cycle of stress hormones and cravings presents one impasse. But more importantly, when your body is excessively acidic, it senses that it is in danger. Therefore, your body is programmed to store fat when acid levels rise in case you will be subsisting on those fat stores. *The Yoga Body Diet* helps restore your natural balance.

why.) The mucus clogs the villi, impairing their ability to draw nutrients from food and send them circulating through your body. So, even if you've been eating a diet that would make Michael Pollan proud, your body hasn't been reaping the benefits. As a result, the brain relays the desperate message to your body to eat more, which gets telegraphed as cravings. Specifically, your brain wants foods brimming with fat because it requires fatty acids to build new cells and feel satiated. Hence, you crave French fries, cheese, and chocolate—not Swiss chard.

But don't stress. While stress is smart, we're smarter. Now that we're minding the body, we can eat and exercise to convey one message: Stop storing fat.

And how fast, you ask? Four weeks, to be exact. Four weeks to clean out your drains and detox your digestive tract. Mark this down in your e-calendar: Five weeks from today, your body will become inhospitable to fat. You'll have a yoga body: long, lean, energized, and ready for the next chapter.

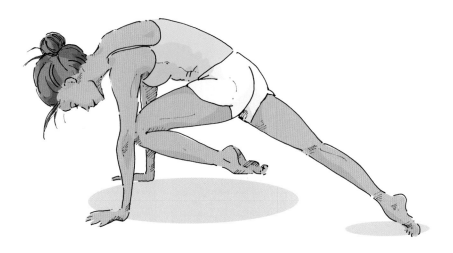

2

THE YOGA BODY DIET: PREVIEW THE PLAN

Whatever it is that pulls the pin, that hurls you past the boundaries
of your own life into a brief and total beauty, even for a moment, it is enough.
—Jeanette

Before we get into the mechanics, here are a few things to keep in mind. First, remember that if the diet feels stressful, you should take a step back. Stop for a day or go back to Week 1. Why? As we mentioned before, stress basically shuts your system down and prevents change and weight loss. This is the opposite of what we're trying to achieve.

If one week you feel derailed by environmental factors (vacation, travel and eating out, long hours at work), just repeat the week. You are probably being too hard on yourself (especially if you are a pitta type, which we'll explain shortly). Yoga emphasizes practice, not perfection. Approach the diet that way.

A second simple guiding principle is that this diet's details are up for interpretation. Yoga and Ayurveda are sciences that are meant to be practiced and prescribed individually. We'd suggest liberating yourself from striving to be the perfect student; invite your creative and interpretive self to play with the recipes and poses. Our philosophy is best embodied by Mark Bittman, the author of the *How to Cook Everything* series, who says in the foreword to his book that he will try to teach the reader to cook like a chef. Chefs use scraps creatively. They interpret recipes rather than following them as if they were law. In *The Yoga Body Diet*, we hope you take our program and make it your own.

Third are the Ayurvedic eating guidelines. In a perfect world, a yogi's place is in the organic kitchen. Outside your window, a vegetable garden would be thriving. We can dream. But getting healthy is coaching yourself to do the best you can with what you have. If you are able to observe the guidelines, do so. If you are stranded in an airport or your personal chef is on vacation, just do your best. Yoga is a practice, not a performance.

Ayurvedic Eating Rules

1. Eat organic. The fewer chemicals your body contends with, the faster it can deal with natural waste products. Plus, you support our land, the farmers who sow it, and an eating style that can sustain our health, our planet, and our progeny.

2. Avoid leftovers. There are many reasons that leftovers are less optimal, including the Indian belief that there is death inside "old" food. We rank this principle so highly because we want to train our taste buds to prefer fresh over fast.

3. "Don't eat standing up, or death looks over your shoulder." This Indian saying underscores the notion that digestion is impaired if you are not relaxed and seated.

4. Don't eat while otherwise occupied. You will eat more if you multitask. In India, eating with your hands remedies the temptation to multitask and therefore cuts down on consuming excess calories.

5. Avoid ice-cold drinks during or after the meal. It's a popular fitness myth to think your body had to work harder to process cold water and you therefore burn more calories. Ayurveda eating considers cold water harder for your body to consume and therefore a stressor.

6. Sip warm or hot water with each meal. Both to stay hydrated and to comfort a hardworking digestive system; sip as you go.

7. Eat until you are satisfied. Yogic eating means being able to stop when your stomach is about three-quarters full. You'll recognize the feeling if you pay attention.

8. Walk. If you can take a short walk after din-ner, you'll feel better, and your food will be absorbed and digested more efficiently.

9. Eat three real meals a day. Skipping meals signals to your body that it may be in danger of missing its food supply. Stave off fat storage by satisfying your body's nutritional and caloric needs three times each day.

10. Eat food according to your type or the sea-son. As a hallmark of this book, you'll learn to eat to balance your specific body type as well as how to eat seasonally, which, simply put, means eat-ing local and organic foods.

No one expects you to be perfect, but we hope at the very least that one day a week you can abide by the rules set forth on the list. However, if you work toward doing the above more often than not, you will find that you can turbocharge your weight loss, and you'll really notice a difference in your health and the taste of your food. Who doesn't favor fresh over last night's fare?

And now, a sneak peak at how to eat.

Preview the Plan

Week 1: Teach Your Body to Burn Fat Again

- *The change:* Change *how,* not *what,* you eat.

- *The benefit:* Hydrate properly, cure cravings, decrease bloating, and eliminate regularly.

During the first week you're going to change *how* you eat. You're going to sip hot water throughout the day. You are going to stop snacking. You're going to aim to eat three to four times a day, making lunch at high noon your heartiest meal. Lastly, you're going to try to eat in peace. No texting, no e-mail, not even talking if you can help it. For those who think this silence sounds impossible, listen to music.

This week reeducates your body to burn fat. Here's how.

1. Ayurveda holds that hot water helps cook up and clear out the gunk in your mucky digestive system. The water is a week-long flushing of the undigested gunk and impurities (that *ama* we mentioned earlier). In our test group, many people stuck to this habit for at least a year after the diet ended, even if they ceased following the other guidelines. Many were happily amazed that all it took to lose weight was a little bit of hot water. Simply being hydrated means your body won't mistake dehydration for hunger.

2. Removing distractions from the eating experience helps you to slow down while eating, which results in achieving greater satisfaction from smaller quantities of food. Mindful eating is a proven weapon against weight gain. Plus, wolfing down lunch and dinner are usually ways of swallowing a lot of stress. If the sandwich is tasteless and lands in the stomach in three heaps, the digestive system doesn't stand a chance.

3. Breathe. The goal here is to stress-proof your body and begin the slim-down process. The simple breathing techniques you'll learn will take 10 minutes a day and will enhance your breath capacity, encourage endurance, and tone your middle. Plus, they will balance your right and left brain, helping you feel calm. We want to tell the nervous system that it doesn't have to worry any more. And it won't take long for the message to get through. According to a National Academy of Sciences study, only 5 days of practicing meditation made students better able to handle stress. Plus, it actively lowered levels of anxiety, depression, anger, and fatigue.

4. Finally, during Week 1, you're also going to take a quiz that reveals your "type." A one-size-fits-all diet fits no one. A hallmark of Ayurveda is its classification of each person as one of three different types, or essences. Ayurveda calls the essences *doshas*. In the West it's common to medicate the symptoms. In the East, the issue is looked at holistically. Knowing your dosha helps you to address your truest self, each remedy is based on balance.

In brief, the types (for that is what we'll call them in the book) are based on three elements we find in nature. You can think of the doshas as personalities, each of which is governed by an element: air, fire, and earth. *Vata* (in Sanskrit) translates to "air"; *pitta* means "fire"; *kapha* is "earth." According to Ayurveda, you get your *dosha* at conception. You have elements of all three, but one is most dominant. When your type is out of balance, you see physical and mental issues. *The Yoga Body Diet* restores balance.

The Yoga Body Diet quiz in the next chapter will help you determine your type and how to eat and move according to principles that will help you maintain balance. We look different from one another, we experience different health issues, we struggle with stress in different ways, and we gain and lose weight differently. Therefore, we require different food and fitness regimens to achieve balance.

Week 2: Eat, Shop, and Cook Yourself Calm

- *The change:* Stop snacking, eat three meals a day, and learn the yoga moves meant for your body type.
- *The benefits:* Reshape your body to be longer and leaner, and cure cravings.

You're going to continue engaging the principles you learned in Week 1, but change *what* you eat based on your type. In Ayurveda, food and yoga are healing. Each type requires foods and poses with different properties in order for you to find balance and lose weight. We've provided the following for each type:

- Shopping list of the best foods
- Yoga moves with unique benefits
- Solutions to common stressors

Why stop snacking? Unlike the grazing habits that we believe destabilize blood sugar, this week's plan pushes your body to feel good on three meals a day. Eating three meals per day without munching in between teaches your body to burn fat both between meals and while you sleep. If you currently feed every 2 to 3 hours, your body never gets a chance to properly break down food (hence, the ama). The constant onslaught of calories makes the body too busy to fully break anything down, eliminate it properly, and keep the blood sugar stable. The blood sugar

spikes and crashes if it's waiting for an injection every 2 hours. Plus, who has time to eat six times a day?

Week 3: Stress-Less Ways to Burn Fat Faster

- *The change:* Shrink dinner, and work out three times a week.
- *The benefit:* Stabilize your blood sugar, and reshape your body with yoga.

"Eat more, weigh less" might be a slogan you've seen before. And it is a sexy come-on; but for the evening meal, less really is more. When we talk about blood sugar in this book, the bottom line is understanding how we end the highs and lows that result in moodiness, cravings, and bad eating habits. Our digestive processes become laden when we send mixed signals. One day the body believes it needs caffeine to produce energy; another day it's chock full of greens and happy. The next day, you're crashing at 4:00 p.m. because you've had no time to eat. By eating three meals, you keep your body happy and your digestion on a tight schedule.

With this new physical component, we go one step further. We make dinner smaller so our bodies have less to deal with as we wind down. Doesn't it make sense to eat the most when digestion peaks, at noon? Dinner gets smaller as a way of further de-stressing the digestive process. A simple supper makes room for the body to process and absorb the meal's nutrients. Plus, less food means fewer calories to process. At night we're winding down anyway, so we don't need energy. We need comfort, sus-

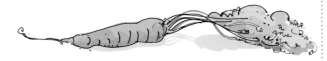

tenance, and the symbolic evening meal; but in Ayurveda it is called a "supplemental" meal—more snack than large meal. The result of eating skinny suppers: We burn fat faster and for a longer stretch of time.

Week 4: Eat, Sleep, and Exercise for All-Day Energy

- *The change:* Eat dinner earlier and practice yoga three times a day.
- *The benefit:* Burn fat while you sleep, and wake up with energy.

There are several reasons why eating a lot before bed will be an issue if you are trying to lose weight. Most importantly, eating late may interrupt your sleep. In an ideal world you would sleep 8 hours, sundown to sunset—and you would dine on farm-raised eggs upon waking. That's not exactly realistic for most people.

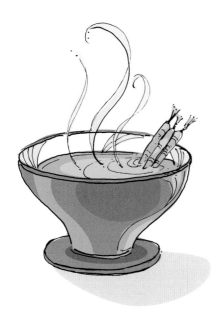

It is worth noting that despite the urge to finish a work project—which might mean you have a snack to get you 2 more hours of computer time—a good night's sleep is worth the investment. "Clean sleep"—8 to 10 hours when your body rests and restores itself as well as cleanses its internal systems—is as critical to your health and well-being as anything else you do. The building blocks of a lifelong way of eating come together in this week. Last week, making dinner smaller made way for more fat burning; making it earlier makes for a better night's sleep. If you can eat, sleep, and exercise your way to an ideal weight, you'll go to bed with good energy, wake up with even more, and never have to worry about a fancy, expensive detoxification at a desert spa. It'll happen nightly. Where formerly you faced sleepless nights and groggy mornings, you'll now feel completely awake and ready for the day. A good night's sleep allows your body to reshape itself, stay relaxed, burn fat, and build muscle. But more importantly, even if you eat well and exercise, without smart sleeping habits, your body's ability to lose weight is not optimized.

You're 4 Weeks Away from a Yoga Body

This plan is not about the yoga. And it's not about Ayurveda. This plan is about you and your connection with your body and mind. Ayurveda and yoga are the food and fitness tools that will reunite you with them.

Let's be realistic. Unless you're planning to sell off your worldly possessions and ship off to an ashram tonight, today's stressors aren't going anywhere. What is going to change is your response to them. Stress will no longer be able to wreak havoc on your body and mind.

For 5,000 years, these ancient Indian prac- tices have healed people and changed their lives. Now the benefits can be yours in just 4 weeks.

Here is a concise chart of the week-by-week plan for easy reference.

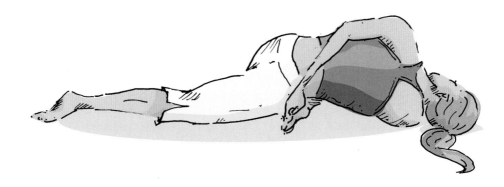

WEEK	BENEFITS	FOOD LESSONS	YOGA PRACTICE	YOUR YOGA BODY DIET TOOLBOX
WEEK 1 **The beginner's guide to building a yoga body**	Re-educate your body to burn fat.	Sip hot water. Eat your biggest meal at noon. Eat mindfully.	De-stress.	1. Do breathing exercises for 10 minutes a day, page 21.
WEEK 2 **Eat, shop, and stretch yourself calm**	Watch cravings disappear.	Eat three meals a day. Stop snacking. Eat and cook for your type.	Do 5 poses from your 20 Power Poses list.	1. Shopping lists for your type, page 36 2. Yoga moves for your type, page 52
WEEK 3 **Healthy habits to burn fat faster**	Stabilize your blood sugar.	Shrink dinner.	Work out. Practice at home three times a week.	30-, 60-, and 90-minute yoga workouts for your type, page 64
WEEK 4 **Eat, sleep, and exercise for all-day energy**	Burn fat faster and longer, especially while you sleep. Wake up with great energy.	Make dinner earlier or skip dinner.	Work out harder.	Skinny supper recipes, page 122
MAINTENANCE **Your yoga body for life**	Become naturally radiant and wholesomely healthy for life.	Eat seasonally. Cleanse twice a year.	Deepen your practice.	1. The 4-day detox 2. Seasonal eating

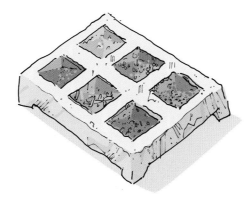

3

WEEK 1: HOW TO EAT RIGHT TONIGHT

Without accepting the fact that everything changes, we cannot find perfect composure.
—Shunryu Suzuki

Part of yoga is being aware of when you are just going through the motions. Maybe you throw your weight around at work or bark orders at your spouse without thinking. Or you hurl your way through the sun salutations like you're doing sprints. One of the most incredible benefits of doing yoga is the ability to evoke and tune into subtle sensations. This attentiveness tends to radiate outward and you're apt to get better results in all areas of your life, including eating.

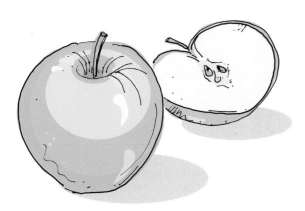

When it comes to eating, because we're in such a rush these days, we usually choke down a sandwich and call that a meal. There's a big trend these days toward "your fat is not your fault" diets that tend to blame our expanding waistlines on everything from an industrialized food supply to hormone imbalance. While those elements are certainly factors, *The Yoga Body Diet* asks you to focus on something you can have an effect on: yourself. On this diet, the first week is about taking some responsibility. Last time we checked, nobody was forcing the fries down your throat while you drove away from the takeout window.

Ayurveda embraces mindful eating by asking you to adjust not *what* you eat, but *how* you eat. This is the easiest way to make an immediate change. Plus, a major diet overhaul would send your nervous system into a frenzy—as any carb- or calorie-starved crabby weight-watcher will attest. Your mantra should be *stress less*. There's no need to memorize food lists or count calories this week. But you should focus on controlling your surroundings when you eat. No matter what the contents of your next meal, you can eat it calmly.

You'll be sipping hot water all day, actively hydrating. You'll also be changing the size and frequency of your meals and making your meals a body and *mind* experience. In this way, the Week 1 fundamentals fire up your body's ability to burn fat without the tools it might have resorted to in the past: stress or starvation. You will lose weight simply by changing *how* you eat the foods you are already eating.

Also think of Week 1 as the quick restart. Holidays, buffets, and vacations are a reality. And if Grandma's southern fried chicken appears on your picnic table once a summer, by all means enjoy it. Try not to stress about eating dinner out; just do your best to order the healthiest option. (Practice, don't perfect.) If mindful eating means that not eating the family's traditional reunion fare will make you irritable and regretful, return to Week 1 to detox after you're done indulging.

The four fundamentals that follow are the best way to reset your health and set yourself up for success on *The Yoga Body Diet.* You can also use these guidelines to rebound from any indulgence.

1. Hydrate with Warm Water

Drinking warm water may seem ridiculously simple, but it is going to be one of the most profound changes you will make. Here's why: 75 percent of Americans are chronically dehydrated. If you're one of them, *congratulations!* This is a good problem to have because it's so easy to remedy. Up to 5 pounds of weight loss is just waiting to happen. Researchers know that in order for your metabolism—the built-in calorie-torcher toiling away 24 hours a day—to work to its fullest potential, your body's cells need to be well hydrated. Just as you feel sluggish when you're parched, your cells—and thus your metabolism—drag when deprived of H_2O.

What's more, a study in the journal *Obesity* shows that replacing sugary beverages like soda and fruit juice with a clear, eco-chic thermos of water automatically reduces the number of calories you consume per day by about 200. Over the course of 1 year, you can shed 21 pounds with almost no effort.

Why must it be warm water? Some diets claim your body burns calories when you drink iced water because your internal systems have to heat the water to meet your internal thermostat. That's perfect if you want to pull the emergency brake on effective digestion. Here's the play-by-play: Cold water causes the muscles and blood vessels in your gastrointestinal tract to freeze. Warm water, on the other hand, relaxes the muscles and dilates the blood vessels. The dilation allows the breakdown (technically called "assimilation") and absorption of the contents of your meal to occur more efficiently. And we now know that any trick that makes stress feel unwelcome means more motivation for the body to get skinny, stat.

According to Ayurveda, warm water is a natural detoxifier. Warm water mops up impurities as it travels through your meandering and—dare we say—overtaxed-for-decades digestive system, sweeping away molecules left behind from partially digested food that could be slowing down what nature intended to be an enviably swift metabolic rate.

When should you sip? Anytime you experience between-meal hunger or cravings, have one or two cups of warm water and wait 10 minutes. If your pangs pass, it may have been thirst. Often, the brain confuses thirst and hunger because the same region, the hypothalamus, detects both. Boil water once or twice during the day and keep it in a large thermos. Electric teakettles and warm water dispensers are easy to find at most offices.

2. Eat Right Now

Mindful eating has a huge impact on how much you eat and how much you weigh. But what does "mindful eating" mean? It's about being conscious and present when you eat. Scientists are discovering that an overwhelming number of factors influence how much you eat on any given day. Everything from your mood and emotions to the color of the walls around you may cause you to eat more or less. Some factors—like how quickly you eat—you can control, while others you can't. (You're not about to have the maître d' raise the lights so you can tally how many steamed mussels are on your plate, are you?)

At the heart of the matter is this: Knowing when you're full requires that all of your senses be present. A single ripe strawberry delivers greater satisfaction when you eat it as if you were tasting a vintage wine in Bordeaux. The reality, however, is that most of us inhale the berry while making a left turn out of the driveway, and we are lucky if we even taste it. In the first scenario, it may take only two or three pieces to achieve satisfaction, while in the slam-dunk session, you've polished off the pint and you're still jonesing for something sweet.

A study in the *British Medical Journal* discovered that people who eat quickly are three times more likely to be overweight than those who take their time. When you invite your senses to a meal (it doesn't take a Buddhist retreat to get them involved), your brain receives the message that you're eating, because it sees, smells, tastes, and feels the food. Your brain then signals your stomach to release the enzymes and juices necessary for digestion. Race through a meal, though, and your brain and stomach hardly recognize that you've eaten. How would they know it's time to stop if you've turned swallowing into yet another life event where you simply go through the motions?

Zoning out while you eat will counteract your efforts to lose weight, not only at the time of your meal but long after. A study in the journal *Appetite* found that ladies who lunched while watching a 10-minute DVD consumed 20 percent more food several hours later compared with those who ate in silence. Researchers believe that the distraction caused the women to forget their meal, so they were hungrier and more easily tempted down the road. Surfing the Internet probably does the same.

According to Ayurveda, you are not only what you eat but *how* you eat. If you eat in haste while under stress, you will undermine the digestive process, which depends on being calm and relaxed to effectively digest. Ayurveda says that

Trick the Coffee Habit

Nonduality is a counterintuitive philosophy associated with yoga. It means that things are neither good nor bad until we label them. Just as stress may be viewed for its positive or negative aspects, so too may our collective caffeine addiction. Coffee certainly has redeeming qualities (including the social aspects); recent studies have found that java may ward off conditions like Alzheimer's and Parkinson's diseases. It may also reduce your risk of skin cancer, gallstones, and diabetes. Researchers attribute coffee's benefits to its boost of antioxidants as well as its caffeine content.

In small amounts, such as a cup after a meal, coffee is a powerful digestive. Being a stimulant, coffee wakes up the intestines and helps food to pass more rapidly through the digestive system.

So drink up, right? Not so fast.

Coffee is highly acidic. This means that it can irritate the intestines, especially when there isn't any food waiting to be digested that can absorb and dilute it. As a result, the acid causes inflammation. The intestine responds by producing a reactive mucus, which, in turn, interferes with our body's ability to absorb nutrients from foods, digest healthily, and detoxify naturally.

Coffee is also dehydrating. Caffeine has a diuretic effect on the body, which means that you urinate more after drinking coffee than when you drink, say, water. If you don't replace the liquid you've lost, then you can easily become dehydrated.

Lastly, as a stimulant, coffee causes the adrenal glands to excrete more cortisol, adrenaline, and epinephrine—the same hormones you release when you're stressed. Although these chemicals keep you awake and alert, these effects are short-lived. When your caffeine levels plummet, you find yourself even more exhausted than you were before your trip to the corner coffee shop and quickly end up in a cycle of *needing* artificial energy to make it through your day. Plus, over time your body acclimates. So, the more you rely on caffeine as a source of energy, the more of it you require to obtain the same energy levels.

Because coffee runs counter to some *Yoga Body Diet* principles, we'd say, if you can't quit, do your best to cut down. One cup a day will keep anxiety at bay. Enjoy the ritual and the taste, and don't be surprised if the bitterness becomes intolerable once your body starts to get what it really needs.

80 percent of all disease starts with digestion, which is challenged by distracted eating and eating on the run. Slow down. Allot at least 20 minutes for each meal. This might have been an unthinkable amount of time when you were eating every 2 hours (for a total of 42 meals a week), but with three meals a day, we are talking about only 1 hour per day. Swear off Twittering, browsing the gossip Web site du jour, booking that hotel, and recasting your to-do list. Even online window shopping can wait. Can't stand the silence? iPods are not contraband. If you have a hard time quieting yourself, make a lunch play list and listen while you eat. We recommend several at www.theyogabodydiet.com. With your attention undivided, you will gain an acute sense of just how much food it takes to fill you up. One hint: It's less than you think.

3. Breathe for Beauty

There is something better for your waistline than a crunch, and it's called a complete breath. What's great about breathing is that even in a boardroom you can do 20 reps of a breathing exercise without looking odd. It's the cheapest and safest workout ever invented. And it can really affect weight loss. Why? The benefits are simultaneously muscular and cerebral.

Your diaphragm is a major muscle that works like an umbrella, opening and closing, with each inhalation and exhalation, over 20,000 times a day. Imagine what we'd look like if we did 20,000 crunches every day. That umbrella action is not only a cardiac massage for the heart, but it also sends fresh air to our oxygen-hungry muscles. If you're tense, your muscles constrict like a boa

around its prey. A deep breath triggers the relaxation response, raising your resistance to stress.

Choose 10 minutes a day to breathe deeply. Can't find an extra second in your busy day? Try appending the 10 minutes to the tail end of something you do every day, like showering or brushing your teeth. If you can't find 10 minutes alone, try it while you wash dishes or drive. Or do the Are You a Chest or Belly Breather exercise on the opposite page first thing in the morning or just before you go to bed. You might start to look thinner after a week of good breathing, because to take a really deep breath, you have to open the chest and draw the shoulder blades down the back.

Each day you can measure your progress by increasing the amplitude of your breath. In other words, if you can extend your breaths for 6 or 7 counts, you'll have increased your lung capacity and endurance and toned your abdominals even in Week 1.

Your nervous system will have a daily reminder that tigers are not chasing you. Breathing exercises also have a soulful benefit. According to yoga, we are all given a finite number of breaths. Observing the breath rather than going through the motions means we are really making them count.

4. Take the Quiz to Find Your Type

The quiz you're about to take is an essential feature of *The Yoga Body Diet*, and it may be unlike anything you've seen before. While this component has been a core concept to Ayurveda practitioners for thousands of years—in fact, guiding everything they do—people often brush it aside

Are You a Chest or a Belly Breather?

Try this: Rest one hand on your abdomen and one hand on your chest. Watch which part of the body rises and falls when you breathe normally. The part that rises highest indicates the type of breather you are.

Most people are either chest or belly breathers. If you use your belly, you constrict your chest, and vice versa.

Our project is to make them both part of the breath. If you're one or the other, chances are you're only at 50 percent of your breath capacity, so you can double your energy and oxygen supply just by recruiting another part of your body to make your breaths deeper. This full breath, sometimes called a three-part breath, is what a baby uses, breathing in its crib—you see both the chest and belly rise and fall steadily. We are aiming to involve the entire body and to equalize the inhale and the exhale. This is the simplest breathing technique—and a form of meditation, if you like.

To practice complete breathing, use this technique 10 minutes a day for the next 5 days.

Full, Complete Breathing

- Sit cross-legged on the floor. (You can also do this in an office chair or while sitting in the car.)
- Switch the foot you put in front to place your "nondominant" ankle in front.
- Touch the backs of your hands to your knees, palms facing skyward.
- Tip your chin down slightly to feel the back of your neck become elongated.
- Exhale firmly to expel all of the oxygen in your belly, cleansing your lungs.
- Turn your eyes to look softly down at your ankles.
- Let your belly become soft and slack.
- Inhale for a count of 5 or 6, visualizing your breath like a warm white light moving from your low abdomen to your mid-belly and up into your chest.
- Exhale for the same count of 5 or 6.

Continue this technique for 10 minutes. At the end of the session, sit quietly and observe the differences in your body and mind. Rub your palms together to create some heat. Drag your palms over your eyes, throat, chest, abdomen, and legs; and finally, rub the bottoms of your feet gently to ground yourself and symbolically seal in some of the energy you just created. As you re-enter your busy life, try to take the sense of calm with you.

as an insignificant aspect to achieving health and irrelevant to losing weight. As you will soon find out, nothing could be more important to accomplishing both goals. It's with great conviction that we believe one diet *doesn't* fit all. Here's how you can determine what kind of diet feels right for your body type—and we don't just mean your build.

It will come as no surprise to learn that weight gain is a symptom of imbalance. Everyday stress, depression, and even the marathon of end-of-year celebrations (no matter how many trips to the spa you take) can catapult you from the calm eye of the storm into the very storm itself. And that, as you know, can send you spelunking for chocolate-covered peanut-butter-filled pretzels and a pint of ice cream at midnight. Every night. Clearly, balance quickly becomes as distant a memory as size 4 jeans.

The distinction between balance and imbalance isn't as obvious as you may think. Balance really means being true to what feels good for you, no matter what external factors are at play. How exactly are you going to do that? It's all about your type, called a *dosha* in Ayurveda.

Your dosha is your essence: your unique arrangement of physical, mental, emotional, and spiritual traits. In short, it's what, from the very beginning, was determined to create your essence. It describes everything from how dry or oily your skin is, to your ability to remember phone numbers, to your preference for hot or cold foods, to the thickness and color of your hair, to whether you work better alone or with others, to your sexual appetite, and so on. There are three doshas: vata, pitta, and kapha. Each shares qualities with an element: vata with air, pitta with fire,

and kapha with earth. You're born with—and need—a combination of all three doshas; but each of us has one dominant dosha. In Sanskrit, this dominant dosha is called your *prakriti*. And that, says Ayurveda, was determined at the moment you were conceived.

When your dominant dosha becomes imbalanced, your physical and emotional health destabilizes, too. Your best quality quickly becomes your worst. For example, a driven and goal-oriented pitta may become as ruthless and as tough on others as she is on herself. A creative vata may become too flighty or overwhelmed to be productive. And a calm, laid-back kapha may allow herself to sleep too much and eat too much and find that her daily routine has her in a rut.

In Ayurveda, food is pacifying, healing, and medicinal. Eating foods that calm your dosha brings your body and mind back into balance. For instance, too much fiery pitta causes symptoms such as inflammation, heartburn, and rash. Emotionally, it can make you quick to anger and competitive. Tempering your fiery side with naturally cooling foods such as fresh mango and juicy cantaloupe recalibrates your system. On the other hand, downing a spicy Mexican meal is akin to dumping gas on an already unrestrained blaze.

Pitta's fire/summer nature requires cooling foods to restore equilibrium. Eating these foods simmers down the excess of fire in the digestive system and makes the body healthier. Similarly, vata's free-flowing air/winter elements need a diet of warm, hearty, oily foods to find terra firma, while kapha's wet earth/spring qualities warrant lighter, drier foods with fiery attributes so it can stop encouraging the calories to stick and start to slough them off.

You may have even followed diets in the past that pushed you more out of whack, thinking they'd help you slim down. For example, a raw-food diet for a dehydration-prone vata is like sucking a desert dry. Getting to the root of who you are and eating foods that help you achieve mind-body balance will make an instant difference in how you look and feel.

The Weight Connection

Simply being in balance will allow your body to easily find its way to what we call its *happy place*—that weight at which you look and feel your absolute best and which you can maintain with minimal effort. You learned in Chapter 1 that a certain amount of stress is essential; it may even be partly responsible for what makes you so vital in the life you've created for yourself. However, too much stress (especially the chronic kind) results in a cascade of hormones and behaviors that encourage your body to cling to—and store—fat.

Each dosha responds uniquely to stress. Vatas may respond with anxiety, insomnia, and irritable bowels; pittas with anger, resentment, and acne; and kaphas with oversleeping, withdrawal, and congestion. While the end result—weight gain—is the same for all, the paths that lead you there differ. Therefore, the tools you engage to dislodge from chronic stress also need to be particular to your dosha.

We've got you covered. You will notice that as your doshic stars align, you begin to feel more "normal" and more like yourself. You'll see your stress levels stay low even when life doesn't go swimmingly. (And let's be honest: How often does it go swimmingly?) In other words, stabilizing your body's chemistry using food and fitness is a simple way to get healthy naturally.

What Is Your Type?

If left to their own devices, pittas would build Rome in a day. Vatas would throw themselves into building Rome, get distracted, and then build some of Verona, but then they'd go back to Rome. Kaphas would labor every day, using well-established rituals, until Rome was built. Where you fit, according to yoga and Ayurveda, depends on your essence.

During this first week, fill out the dosha questionnaire on the following pages. For each item, circle the answer that most accurately describes how you are right now. If two answers apply, circle both. If none applies, leave it blank. Then, tally your A's, B's, and C's. The letter you circled most is your dominant dosha. The second most frequent answer indicates that you also possess many of that dosha's qualities, while the least frequent plays a lesser role in describing who you are.

Without further ado, here's the quiz.

The Yoga Body Diet Quiz:

What's Your Type?

Describe your mental activity.
A. Quick mind; restless
B. Sharp intellect; aggressive
C. Calm, steady, stable

Describe your memory.
A. Short-term is best
B. Good general memory
C. Long-term is best

Your thoughts are:
A. Constantly changing
B. Fairly steady
C. Steady, stable, fixed

Describe your concentration.
A. Short-term focus is best
B. Better-than-average focus
C. Long-term focus is best

Describe your learning style.
A. Quick grasp of learning
B. Medium to moderate grasp
C. Slow to learn new things

Describe your dreams.
A. Fearful; involve running, flying, jumping
B. Angry, fiery, violent, adventurous
C. Include water, clouds, relationships, romance

Your sleep is:
A. Interrupted, light
B. Sound, medium
C. Sound, heavy, long

Your speech is:
A. Fast, sometimes missing words
B. Fast, sharp, clear-cut
C. Slow, clear, sweet

Your voice is:
A. High pitched
B. Medium pitched
C. Low pitched ·

Your eating speed is:
A. Quick
B. Medium
C. Slow

Your hunger levels are:
A. Irregular
B. Sharp; need food when hungry
C. Can easily miss meals

Describe your food and drink preferences.
A. Prefer warm
B. Prefer cold
C. Prefer dry and warm

Describe your approach to achieving goals.
A. Easily distracted
B. Focused and driven
C. Slow and steady

You give and donate:
A. Small amounts
B. Nothing or large amounts infrequently
C. Regularly and generously

Describe your relationships.
A. Many casual
B. Intense
C. Long and deep

Your sex drive is:
  A. Variable or low
  B. Moderate
  C. Strong

You work best:
  A. While supervised
  B. Alone
  C. In groups

Describe your weather preference.
  A. Aversion to cold
  B. Aversion to heat
  C. Aversion to damp, cool

Describe your reaction to stress.
  A. Excite quickly
  B. Medium
  C. Slow to get excited

Financially, you:
  A. Don't save; spend quickly
  B. Save, but spend big
  C. Save regularly; accumulate wealth

Your friendships:
  A. Tend toward short-term;
  make friends quickly
  B. Tend to last longer; friends are related to
  occupation
  C. Tend to be long-lasting

Your moods:
  A. Change quickly
  B. Change slowly
  C. Are steady, unchanging

You react to stress with:
  A. Fear
  B. Anger
  C. Indifference

In an argument, you are most sensitive to:
  A. Your own feelings
  B. No one; not sensitive
  C. Others' feelings

When threatened, you tend to:
  A. Run
  B. Fight
  C. Make peace

Your relationship with your partner/spouse is:
  A. Clingy
  B. Jealous
  C. Secure

You express affection:
  A. With words
  B. With gifts
  C. With touch

When feeling hurt you:
  A. Cry
  B. Argue
  C. Withdraw

Describe your most common emotional trauma.
  A. Anxiety
  B. Denial
  C. Depression

Describe your confidence level.
  A. Timid
  B. Outwardly self-confident
  C. Inner confidence

The amount of hair you have is:
  A. Average
  B. Thinning
  C. Thick

Your hair type is:

A. Dry

B. Normal

C. Oily

Your (natural) hair color is:

A. Light brown or blonde

B. Red or auburn

C. Dark brown or black

Your skin type is:

A. Dry, rough, or both

B. Soft, normal to oily

C. Oily, moist, cool

Describe your skin temperature.

A. Cold hands/feet

B. Warm

C. Cool

Your complexion is:

A. Darker

B. Pink, red

C. Pale, white

Your eyes are:

A. Small

B. Medium

C. Large

The whites of your eyes are:

A. Bluish brownish

B. Yellow or red

C. Glossy white

The size of your teeth is:

A. Very large or very small

B. Medium-small

C. Medium-large

Describe your usual weight.

A. Thin; hard to gain

B. Medium

C. Heavy; gain easily

Naturally your daily elimination is:

A. Dry, hard, thin; easily constipated

B. Frequent during the day, soft to normal

C. Heavy, slow, thick, regular

Your veins and tendons are:

A. Very prominent

B. Fairly prominent

C. Well covered

Your natural exercise tolerance is:

A. Low

B. Medium

C. High

Without training, your endurance is:

A. Fair

B. Good

C. Excellent

Without training, your strength is:

A. Fair

B. Better than average

C. Excellent

In a footrace, your speed is:

A. Very good

B. Good

C. Not so fast

With friends and family, you:

A. Don't like competitive pressure

B. Are a driven competitor

C. Deal easily with competitive pressure

On your way in to buy a coffee, your walking speed is:

A. Fast

B. Average

C. Slow

With or without a fitness program, your muscle tone is:

A. Lean, low body fat

B. Medium with good definition

C. Brawny or bulky, with higher fat percentage

Describe your body size as it relates to buying clothes.

A. Small frame; lean or long (bird-like, petite shopper)

B. Medium frame (shoulders and arm length fit most clothing off the rack without alterations)

C. Large frame; fleshy (may go up one size and alter the length)

If someone throws keys for you to catch, how fast is your reaction?

A. Quick

B. Average

C. Slow

TALLY YOUR TYPE

Count how many A's, B's, and C's you selected throughout the questionnaire.

A's _____

B's _____

C's _____

Key: A = Vata B = Pitta C = Kapha

4

WEEK 2: EAT, SHOP, AND STRETCH YOURSELF CALM

I felt emotions of gentleness and pleasure that had long appeared dead, revive within me.
—Mary Shelley

So far you've learned how yoga and Ayurveda are going to help you lose weight while reining in stress and giving hunger the boot. You'll be happy to learn that this week is about getting personal. The diet and exercise plan is customized to you. This week you're going to gain vital insight into who you are by learning more about your *prakriti,* or dominant dosha. Here's where the pounds begin to fall off, because you're going to buy, eat, and cook foods that temper your dosha. Instead of giving your body what you think it wants, you're going to be feeding it exactly what it needs.

Here are this week's fundamentals.

1. STOP SNACKING AND EAT THREE MEALS A DAY

We love snacks as much as you do. But we've got some bad news: Grazing can lead to weight gain.

How? Frequent meals destabilize your blood sugar because you become reliant on the 2-hour cycle: eating and crashing, eating and crashing. Because your body learns to expect food every 2 to 3 hours, your blood sugar spikes and dips just as quickly. The result? You're famished and slumped over with fatigue—*all day long.* (Sound familiar?) The stress test applies again: Who has time to plan 42 perfectly healthy meals every week? Not to mention the fact that a "saintly" 200- to 300-calorie meal is barely enough to keep you energized until the next feeding anyway.

The six-meals-a-day concept can stall weight loss in yet another way. The constant intake of food prevents your body from burning its own fat because you're providing it with fuel almost around the clock.

The Yoga Body Diet re-educates your body to burn fat by going back to the basics: Eat three meals per day. By learning to burn stored fat between meals and especially overnight, your fat cells stop clinging for dear life to the nearest calorie. You stop the body's and the brain's belief that you've switched to a pattern of deprivation. You may be very familiar with restrictions and the hippo-sized hunger that results. But hunger has no place in this plan. Hunger is stressful.

How, then, is it possible to go from breakfast to lunch and lunch to dinner without sneaking a snack or feeling like you cheated? The answer is eating three large, delicious, satisfying meals every day. We encourage you to experiment at first with a little trial and error. For instance, if you crash at 4:00 p.m., then you can safely say your lunch was too small. If you are feeling low on energy because your bento box was insufficient at noon, have a snack that will tide you over until dinner. Some suggestions? Nuts and dried fruits are perfect go-to foods. The portion is about a handful.

Use this experience and information to gain insight about your body. Remember: *The Yoga Body Diet* is about reconnecting your body and mind, not muscling through starvation. You may discover that tomorrow you simply need to eat more food at lunch. Don't feel bad about the snacking. You didn't violate the rule; you simply learned that your body needs more food to make it from one meal to the next.

Use the sample meal plan below, which you can use anytime, anywhere. If you have to order out or you're traveling, eating as close to this plan as possible will keep you on track.

Now that you know your type, try to include foods meant to pacify your dosha. In Chapter 8, you'll find recipes that capitalize on the ingredients that will help you to achieve balance. In the back of the book, you'll find a day-by-day, week-by-week plan if you like to cook at home.

What Three Meals a Day Looks Like

Breakfast

- Fruit
- Hot cereal
- Toast and herbal tea

Lunch

- Salad or soup
- Veggies
- Rice or pasta
- Chicken or tofu
- Dessert with herbal tea

Dinner

- Soup or salad
- Fruit
- Sandwich
- Small dessert with herbal tea

2. Learn About Your Type So You Can Eat Right

What do you do when you've discovered whether you are a vata, pitta, or kapha? The answer: Eat! The next three sections are divided by type, each dedicated to one dosha, like your personal owner's manual. Here's what you will find:

• Your type profile: A complete description of your dosha's physical, mental, and spiritual characteristics

• Your shopping list: A categorized list of the foods that balance your type

You don't need us to list the health and weight-loss virtues of cooking versus eating away from home. You are probably already well aware of what happens to your body when you forego homemade meals in favor of sugar-, salt-, and grease-laden restaurant fare. Plus, let's face it: Your favorite eatery doesn't give a hoot whether their dishes are dosha-friendly.

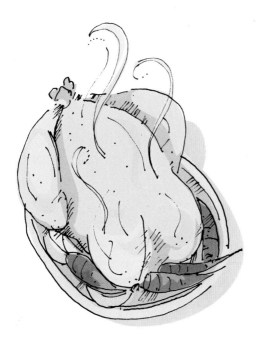

These are just a few reasons why one of the most significant changes you can make, if you haven't made it already, is preparing your meals yourself. There is also a deeply spiritual (or at the very least, relaxing) quality to cooking your own food. Remember, even dicing carrots fulfills the criteria set forth by Dr. Herbert Benson for activities that elicit the relaxation response. Cooking involves many repetitive actions (stirring, chopping, peeling, and so on). It encourages you to set aside intruding thoughts because following a recipe requires concentration and carefulness.

We created recipes (Chapter 8) in the tradition of spa food: fresh ingredients, quick preparation, and delicious flavors that satisfy all of your senses. They are also budget-, earth-, and vegetarian-friendly. (Although they include lean proteins such as fish and chicken, you can easily use tofu, tempeh, seitan, and other substitutes.) We also tried to ensure that despite the Ayurvedic rules, these meals are realistic. This means that they are simple, fresh, and dinner party worthy. What we wound up with was a menu that will have you healthy in no time. And it doesn't require a culinary degree, either.

Over the next 7 days, you are going to eat very well. Because we've asked you to cut out snacks, the meals need to be big and filling to sustain you from one meal to the next. And they are. This means you're going to be eating like a (svelte) queen, not a scavenging chipmunk. Maybe the best news of all is that you don't have to count a single calorie. And you don't have to figure out which ingredients to use in order to balance your dosha. Although the dishes are the same for everyone (Tea-Poached Chicken, Veggie Soufflé, and Pad

Thai, to name a few) there are three versions of each recipe—vata, pitta, and kapha—that use only the ingredients you need and none of those you don't.

When it comes to eating this week, turn to Chapter 8 and select any breakfast, any lunch, and any dinner that you want to eat each day. (If you're like us, you know that deciding what to eat is half the battle, and we've made it incredibly easy for you!) Then, follow the recipe for your dosha and dig in (in a serene, mindful manner, of course).

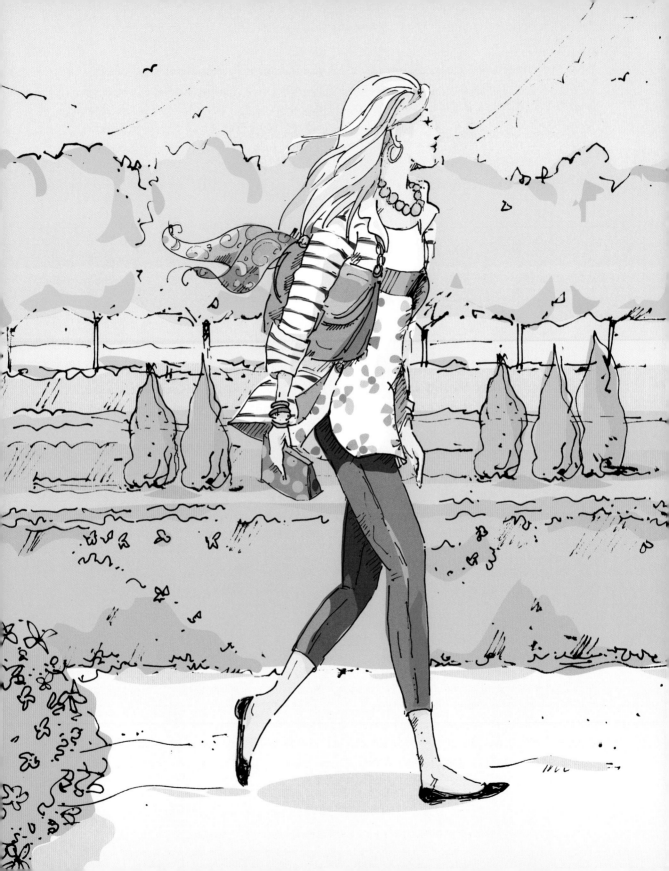

VATA

Airy in nature

*It had the effect of a spell, taking her out of the ordinary relations
with humanity and enclosing her in a sphere by herself.*
—Nathaniel Hawthorne

Nervous? Anxious? Restless? You blame these familiar feelings on your stressful job, rocky relationship, or predilection for caffeine in every form. Wrong! It's your dosha. Stressors like a lack of sleep or an impending deadline can send vata spiraling into worry, anxiety, fatigue, and depression. These feelings often become distracting and keep you from accomplishing anything. But it's not all grim. A balanced vata is creative, artistic, sensitive, spiritual, and funny. You just need to find your way back to, well, you! Follow our food and fitness roadmap, and you'll do even better. You'll learn how to stay there.

Vata is associated with air and winter. Imagine a frigid wind ripping through a field on a brisk January morning. Its speed and direction change suddenly and without warning, as do you. You've likely had more relationships, careers, hobbies, and dress sizes than you care to count. Similarly, vatas are indecisive, and your mood and mind can turn on a dime. Your predominant physical qualities are cold and dry. You're constantly seeking warmth, and because coldness cannot maintain moisture, your skin is often dry, dull, and flaky.

THE WEIGHT FACTOR

Vatas are the ultimate grazers, mostly because they lack the order and routine necessary for planning meals. Keep in mind that the all-day-eating trend caught on like wildfire because we live in a culture that in many ways is vata: fast-paced, overloaded, and unpredictable. But as you will soon find out, grazing (regardless of whether it's on corn chips or seaweed crackers) backfires because your body never gets a chance to burn its own fat for fuel. Eating three meals a day, however, will quickly turn your body into a well-oiled fat-burning machine.

Vatas also experience an irregular appetite; on some days you could down the entire contents of your pantry, while on other day you get by on a few carrot sticks here, a handful of M&M's there. Creating the time to enjoy three daily meals will yield major returns. First, it will put your appetite on a more predictable schedule so you don't wind up drooling over a fat- and sugar-laden calorie bomb at the nearest coffee joint. Second, mealtime will become an oasis in your hectic day as you establish this routine. The structured, dependable activity of eating (as opposed to something that occurs randomly or while stuck in rush hour traffic) relaxes your nervous system and annihilates stress as you nourish your body and your mind. And third, eating in this serene state (i.e., sitting at a table) will enable you to digest your meal properly, in turn reducing the common vata complaint of constipation, caused by eating sporadically and on the run.

THE VATA DIET

Vata's cold and dry disposition requires just the opposite to achieve balance: a high-fat, high-protein diet that is satisfying, lubricating, and grounding. Here is a glance at just some of the ways in which the vata diet will bring you into balance.

Vata imbalance: Anxiety and depression
The fix: Fatty acids

Ayurveda prescribes a high-fat, high-protein diet for those suffering from anxiety and depression, typical symptoms of a vata imbalance. Now, twenty-first-century science is confirming that foods like nuts, fish, and oils contain nutrients that mollify these imbalances. One recent study, published in the journal *Nutrition*, tracked the moods and diets of more than 3,000 women over 20 years and reported that those who consumed the highest doses of the omega-3 polyunsaturated fatty acids (from sources such as salmon and walnuts—both vata-diet approved) had the lowest risk of depression. Good thing, because new research in the journal *Psychosomatic Medicine* found that depressed women carry 25 percent more belly fat than those who are not depressed. And, a study by the University of Pittsburgh School of Medicine found that a diet rich in fatty acids counters depression, negativity, and—wait for it—impulsiveness. Clearly, Eastern and Western science agree that adequate fat is essential for balancing vata.

Vata imbalance: Dryness
The fix: Oils

No oil is off limits in the vata diet. In addition to their mood-boosting qualities, oils (and oil-rich foods) moisturize from the inside out. Besides having dry skin and cracked lips, vatas also experience stiff joints only the Tin Man could understand. An oily diet combined with yoga postures such as Forward Folds that send blood, fluid, and oxygen rushing to your muscles and joints will soothe stiffness and prevent more serious conditions, like arthritis, from developing.

One of the most important guidelines for balancing vata is to eat the majority of foods warm. A bowl of cold cereal with cold milk serves you in no way. However, the fats, protein, and heat in a mug of steaming minestrone soup are just what the Ayurveda doctor ordered.

Vata Superfoods

Beets

These vegetables are sweet and rich in vitamin A. They soothe and protect the mucous membranes (perfect for vatas, who tend to experience dryness).

Sweet potatoes

A sweet, heavy, and warm root vegetable, the sweet potato is great for vata body types.

Dates

These dried fruits are warm and heavy, making a great food—and snack, when you absolutely need it—for vata. They're high in copper, which helps iron absorption while soothing the gut, calming the mind, and rejuvenating the body.

Eggs

As a high-quality complete protein source, eggs offer a wonderful alternative to meat. Since they are sweet and warm and mostly protein and fat, they're ideal for vata body types.

Papayas

Papayas are abundant in natural digestive enzymes.

Amaranth

This high-protein, gluten-free grain is best for vata types because of its heavy and warm properties.

Fennel

Fennel is a balancing vegetable that is calming for the mind and strengthening for the digestive system.

Freshwater fish

High in essential fatty acids and proteins, freshwater fish are excellent for vata types. Plus, their high oil content is nourishing to dry skin.

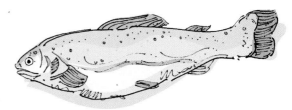

Figs

Figs are purifying for the intestines, liver, and kidneys.

Mangoes

Native to India, this fruit is sweet, slightly sour, and warm. Mangoes are a tonic for the nervous system and intestinal tract.

THE VATA DIET GUIDELINES

- Choose high-protein foods such as nuts, chicken, turkey, meat, and fish.

- Increase use of oils in cooking.

- Favor warm foods; avoid cold and dry foods.

When you're in the grocery store staring at the bulk bin of brown rice, you'll want to know whether this food fits the bill and will temper your vata dosha to help you lose weight. (The answer is yes.) That's why we devised this grocery list to stock your kitchen with the absolute best foods for vata. Copy and post it on your refrigerator, or leave it in your car so you always have it on hand.

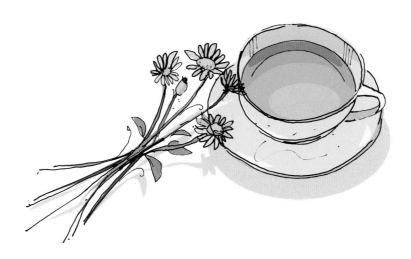

*Favor these Foods

VEGETABLES

Artichokes
Beets*
Brussels sprouts*
Carrots*
Eggplant—cooked
Garlic*
Hot chili peppers
Leeks
Okra
Onions
Parsley
Potatoes
Pumpkins*
Seaweed
Squash—acorn
Squash—winter*
Sweet potatoes*
Tomatoes*
Turnips

FRUITS

Apples, cooked
Apricots
Blueberries
Cantaloupe
Cherries
Coconuts
Cranberries
Dates*
Figs*
Grapefruit*
Grapes*
Guava
Lemons*
Limes*
Mangoes*
Nectarines

Oranges*
Papayas*
Peaches
Pears—ripe
Persimmons*
Pineapples
Strawberries
Tangerines*

SPICES AND HERBS

Anise*
Asafetida*
Basil*
Bay leaf
Black pepper*
Caraway
Cardamom*
Cayenne
Chamomile
Cinnamon*
Clove
Coriander
Cumin*
Dill
Fennel*
Fenugreek
Garlic
Ginger*
Horseradish
Marjoram
Mustard
Nutmeg
Oregano
Peppermint
Rosemary
Saffron*
Sage
Spearmint

Thyme
Turmeric*

LEGUMES

Mung—split yellow
Tofu

NUTS AND SEEDS

Almonds—raw, soaked*
Filberts*
Flaxseeds*
Pine nuts*
Poppy seeds
Sunflower seeds

MEATS AND FISH

Chicken*
Eggs (in moderation)
Freshwater fish*
Saltwater fish*

CONDIMENTS

Mayonnaise—reduced fat
Pickles
Salt
Vinegar

OILS (for cooking only)

Almond
Avocado
Canola
Coconut
Chili peppers*
Corn
Olive
Safflower
Sesame

DAIRY AND DAIRY SUBSTITUTES

Butter
Buttermilk
Cottage cheese*
Ghee*
Milk—not cold
Rice milk
Soy milk
Yogurt

GRAINS

Amaranth*
Brown rice*
Oats*
Quinoa*
Wheat*

BEVERAGES

Water (warm or hot)

HERBAL TEAS

Cardamom*
Chamomile*
Cinnamon*
Cloves*
Ginger*
Orange peel*

SWEETENERS
(in moderation)

Honey—raw
Maple syrup
Molasses
Sugar—raw
Rice syrup

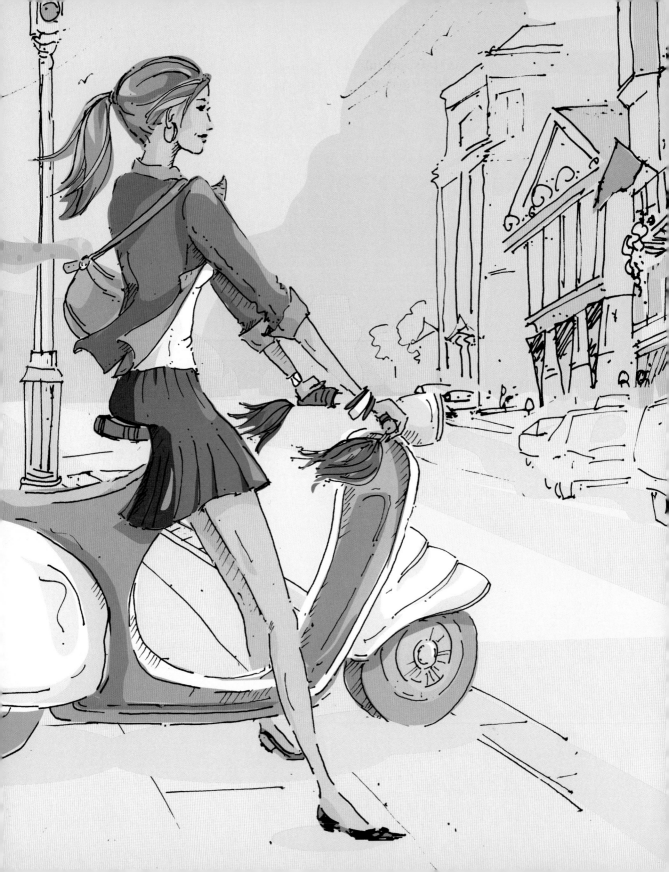

PITTA

Fiery in nature

Her sound opinions and good sense, her shrewd answers and her general behavior,
have won her universal esteem and compliments. . . .
—Jean-Jacques Rousseau

Driven, competitive, and ambitious, you're constantly chasing after your next goal. Typically described as type A's, pittas are extremely intelligent and possess laser-sharp focus. You gravitate toward experiences that test the very limits of your abilities, whether that means running a marathon, earning *another* degree, or spearheading a successful business venture. That doesn't exactly mean you're reckless or thrill-seeking; a pitta's moves are carefully calculated to yield success.

Pittas are known for being well-acquainted with anger. When stressed, your fuse is short, especially in situations where you feel a loss of control—or when you're over-caffeinated. You are as aggressive about calming down as you are about reaching your goals. Your fiery nature can also lead to cyclical burnout because you thrive on the kind of intensity that is nearly impossible to sustain.

When your pitta essence is too strong, your fire and summer qualities result in inflammatory conditions such as rashes, ulcers, irritable bowel syndrome, and high blood pressure. Don't stress. On the pitta diet, you will be cool as a cucumber (which, by the way, is pitta's best vegetable for balance) without losing your edge. Your edge will just become a little less lethal and a little more loving.

THE WEIGHT FACTOR

Hunger for pitta is intense. If you go too long without eating and your blood sugar levels plummet, you experience lightheadedness and irritability. But here's the catch: Pittas frequently forget to eat or can't afford to stop what they're doing to consume something healthy. Those people you see in the elevator at 3 p.m., starving because they are just going to lunch—typical pittas. You become so absorbed in your day that before you know it, the sun has set and you're still running on the energy bar you inhaled that morning on your way out the door. But that means you're trucking on fewer calories, the perfect recipe for weight loss, right? Not so much. As any famished and undernourished pitta can attest, deprivation leads to disaster: scarfing down whatever's near, which is often oily and acidic. Pizza or similarly spicy, fatty foods offer immediate gratification for pittas grabbing a bite.

As if that weren't enough to hinder even the best waist-whittling intentions, your body quickly adapts to the cycle of feast and famine by storing fat. Instead of burning off the ill-advised extra-hot calzone, your body finds a home for it on your belly, hips, and thighs and hangs on to it for dear life. What's more, when you're starving, the body craves fuel in its most rapidly digestible form: sugar. Because a doughnut is digested as quickly as it is consumed, you're constantly seeking your next rush. It's not a happy, healthy, or helpful cycle to be in, especially when it comes to weight loss. And this is criminal abuse for your blood sugar. It is common for the pitta cycle to be full of cravings, and because pittas are goal oriented, the craving is instantly gratified with ample sugar or caffeine. Sound familiar?

What's worse is that you might have previously been able to get away with this kind of unwise eating because your body was thin for the early part of your life. But soon enough, pitta bodies begin to pack it on. One pitta plus: Research says they have the fastest success in pulling off pounds.

The Yoga Body Diet principles are going to provide tremendous relief for the alpha-stressed pitta. The three-meals-a-day regimen that follows will instantly check the swings in your blood sugar and your moods. (Your coworkers and children will thank us.) Having your largest meal in the middle of the day will provide your body and brain with the fuel they

need to perform at the level you demand of them. Lastly, the warm water habit will control the sugar and spice cravings that pittas are prone to as well.

THE PITTA DIET

Whether it's anger, eczema, or heartburn they're dealing with, pittas need to chill, inside and out. Ayurveda's answer? A diet that favors naturally cooling foods (thanks to high water content), such as mangoes and broccoli, while avoiding those that stoke the fire, like the spicy and salty Mexican fare that may be a staple for the hot food lover. The pitta diet also features slowly digested carbohydrates, such as those found in barley, and belly-filling fiber from beans and legumes. Here are two specific ways the pitta diet brings your body back into balance.

Pitta imbalance: Inflammation
The fix: Plant foods and fiber

The real issue for pitta is inflammation caused by an excess of heat. Chronic inflammation, which may be caused by chronic stress, has been linked to a slew of diseases, such as diabetes, high blood pressure, cancer, and heart disease. Perhaps these aren't your greatest health threats at the moment, but they may be down the road. Flare-ups might be festering without your knowing. Or you may have had other inflammatory conditions, such as heartburn or rashes. A pitta-pacifying diet is your antidote. Studies have found that antioxidants, naturally occurring compounds in fruits and vegetables, reduce inflammation. Whole grains such as oats, barley, and wheat—all pitta-diet approved—do, too. Pennsylvania State University researchers recently found that increasing whole grain intake resulted in lower blood levels of a

Pitta Superfoods

Asparagus

This vegetable possesses the qualities of bitterness, sweetness, and astringency—all features that balance pitta. It is a diuretic that helps cleanse the blood and kidneys.

Apples

All varieties are cooling and cleansing for pitta. The apple pectin cleans the gut, and the sweet and astringent aspect of the apple cools the liver and the blood.

Blueberries

These berries are sweet and astringent and known to clean the blood, move the lymph, and balance blood sugar levels, which are all needed to protect pitta types from inflammation.

Cabbage

Loaded with minerals and high in vitamins C and A, cabbage is traditionally used for skin conditions, ulcers, and inflammation.

Celery

This highly alkaline food flushes the lymph and blood, which helps to cool a pitta.

Dandelion

This edible flower is a natural diuretic that flushes the blood and kidneys while providing high amounts of potassium and vitamin A to replenish the body from the effects of its diuretic and cleansing properties.

Grapes

They're sweet, cooling, and high in magnesium. They also cool a pitta and combat inflammation.

Guava

High in vitamin C, guava is a tropical fruit with cooling properties.

Pineapples

This tropical fruit contains natural anti-inflammatory enzymes.

Tofu

The soybean is very high in protein and is easier to digest than other beans.

marker of inflammation called C-reactive protein. In the same study, obese adults who upped their daily whole grain quota also shed more belly fat than those who continued eating refined grains.

It all comes down to fiber. While fiber is also a major player in the vata and kapha diets, it makes a huge appearance in the pitta diet. That's because the pitta diet is largely plant-based (emphasizing fruits, vegetables, whole grains, legumes, and beans), and plants are the richest sources of fiber. Fiber binds with liquids to form a gel as it slowly passes through your digestive system, keeping you feeling fuller longer. One recent study found that women who doubled their fiber intake absorbed 90 fewer calories per day. That's more than 9 pounds lost over the course of a year just by making a few extra stops at the farm stand.

Studies have also found that increasing fiber intake is incredibly valuable for those suffering from irritable bowel syndrome. A common condition when pitta is too strong, irritable bowel syndrome is characterized by alternating bouts of constipation and diarrhea as well as severe abdominal cramping, bloating, and gas. Boosting fiber to the recommended level of 25 grams per day adds bulk to stool while also allowing it to pass more gingerly through your system.

Pitta imbalance: Excess heat and heartburn
The fix: Avoiding most spices

In addition to choosing cooling, water- and fiber-rich foods, avoid spices as much as possible. Spices stoke the pitta fire, but you're looking to squelch it. Think about how you feel after downing spicy Buffalo wings, chili, or fajitas. Your face is red, you're sweating, and you're rummaging around the medicine cabinet for antacids. In other words, you just doused your fire with rocket fuel. Luckily, your beloved spice rack isn't contraband. You just have to move the chili peppers to your kapha pal's counter and bring coriander, mint, cardamom, and fennel to the forefront to reap their cooling qualities.

THE PITTA DIET GUIDELINES

- Eat cooling foods such as fresh fruits and vegetables, dairy, beans, and grains.

- Avoid spicy, salty foods.

THE PITTA SHOPPING LIST

Navigate any supermarket with this shopping list to stock up on pitta-pacifying foods. Copy and post it on your refrigerator, or leave it in your car or office so you always have it on hand.

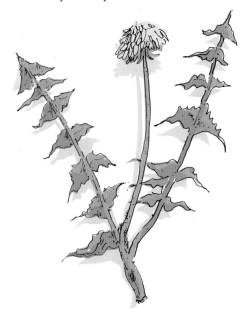

*Favor these Foods

VEGETABLES

Alfalfa sprouts
Artichokes*
Asparagus*
Bean sprouts
Beet greens*
Broccoli*
Cabbage*
Cauliflower*
Celery*
Collard greens
Corn
Cucumbers*
Dandelion*
Eggplant
Endive
Fennel*
Green beans
Jicama*
Kale*
Lettuce*
Mushrooms
Mustard greens
Okra*
Pumpkin
Radishes
Seaweed*
Spinach
Squash, acorn*
Squash, winter
Sweet potatoes
Swiss chard
Tomatoes
Turnip greens
Watercress*
Zucchini*

FRUITS

Apples*
Apricots*
Avocado
Blueberries*
Cantaloupe*
Cherries (ripe)*
Dates
Dried fruit
Figs
Grapes*
Guavas*
Mangoes*
Melon (all)*
Nectarines
Oranges
Papayas
Peaches (ripe and/or peeled)*
Pears*
Persimmons*
Pineapples*
Plums*
Pomegranates*
Raspberries*
Strawberries*
Tangerines

SPICES AND HERBS

Anise
Asafetida
Cardamom
Chamomile*
Cilantro*
Cinnamon
Coriander*
Cumin
Fennel
Ginger
Parsley
Peppermint
Saffron
Spearmint

LEGUMES

Adzuki*
Bean sprouts
Black gram*
Fava*
Garbanzo*
Kidney
Lentils
Lima
Mung*
Peas
Snow peas*
Split peas*
Tofu*

NUTS AND SEEDS

Coconut*
Flax
Pumpkin*
Sunflower*

MEATS AND FISH

Chicken
Eggs (in moderation)
Freshwater fish

CONDIMENTS

Mayonnaise—reduced-fat

OILS (for cooking only)

Coconut
Olive
Soy
Sunflower
Ghee

DAIRY AND DAIRY SUBSTITUTES

Butter
Cottage cheese
Ghee*
Rice milk
Soy milk*

GRAINS

Barley*
Oats
Rice*
Wheat (in moderation)
(Do not eat bread with yeast.)

BEVERAGES

Water (warm)

HERBAL TEA

Chicory*
Hibiscus*
Mint*

SWEETENERS

Maple syrup
Raw sugar
Rice syrup

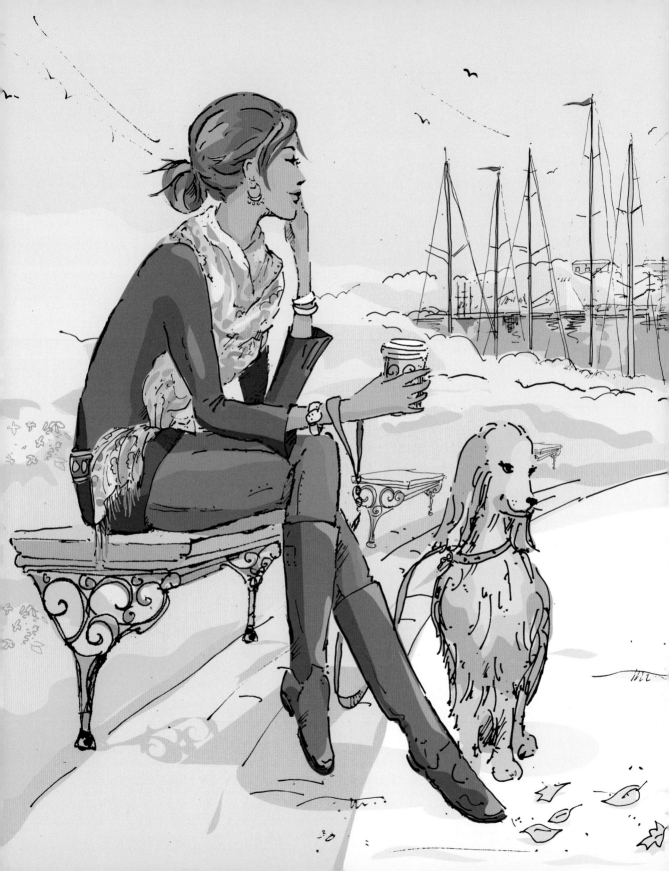

KAPHA

Earthy in nature

All the being and doing, expansive, glittering, vocal, evaporated;
and one shrunk, with a sense of solemnity, to being oneself. . . .
—Virginia Woolf

Kapha types move through life at a slow, methodical pace. Even as the world buzzes around you, you remain calm, easygoing, and generally content. You're warm and generous with your emotions, and you make a loving and loyal partner. You've had the same friends for as long as you can remember, thanks to your capacity and preference for deep and lasting relationships. You bask in order and routine and adapt to change gradually and often begrudgingly.

Your groundedness does not make you immune to imbalance, however. True, kaphas are less likely to get swept up in chaos than vatas or pittas (mostly because you react to stress more slowly than others), but you still enter the storm from time to time. Kaphas react to tension by retreating and ritualizing. Here's what this looks like: hours of intimacy with your couch and your flat screen, oversleeping, and lethargy. Your spring-like qualities mean you build up an excess of moisture in the form of mucus and phlegm in the lungs and sinuses,

increasing your propensity for the congestive condition du jour: allergies, asthma, and other respiratory issues.

All doshas gain weight when they are out of balance, but kaphas tend to have a more difficult time losing it because their bodies naturally want to cling to what they accrue. In no way does this mean that you're headed for a wardrobe of elastic-waist pants. It does, however, explain why one-size-fits-all diets have been especially unsuccessful for you. The kapha diet is specially designed to encourage your body to release the water and weight it's been storing while giving your metabolism the jumpstart it needs. And, by bringing your mind and body into balance, the diet will prevent you from stockpiling stress.

THE WEIGHT FACTOR

We're willing to bet that you already eat three meals per day (or at least try to) because it's a routine, and kaphas love a neat and orderly schedule.

Now that you know the benefits of eating thrice-daily meals and putting the kibosh on snack time, we encourage you to put the extra effort into making your regular mealtime intentions daily realities. The most significant change you'll make to this habit you already have is choosing foods that balance your dosha instead of those that foster sluggishness.

When it comes to weight loss, your yoga practice is going to benefit you in ways that are distinct from those designed for vata and pitta. The other doshas require practices that are gradual and grounding, with longer holds, deeper twists, and restorative folds. Vata and pitta will achieve balance and weight loss by slowing their erratic nervous systems. The kapha practices, however, are designed to amp you up. Imbalance causes kapha to succumb to physical inactivity and a general inertia. In other words, your tendency is to throw a welcome party for unwanted pounds. Kapha's yoga sessions are packed with Sun Salutations, energizing back bends, and vinyasas (literally, *vinyasa* means "flow," where one pose transitions into the next) to increase your heart rate and torch calories. This increase in activity will also boost metabolism, so your body burns, instead of stores, what it consumes.

THE KAPHA DIET

An out-of-balance kapha is inclined to reach for heavier foods, such as ice cream or French fries, that provide a sense—no matter how fleeting—of security and comfort. These are qualities that you naturally possess in abundance when in balance but which you seek outside yourself when unable to summon them from within. Instead, the kapha diet is centered around low-calorie, low-fat foods. We hesitate to use these terms because, from experience, you hear them and think zero-flavor diet fare—cardboard—and starvation. The difference is that most low-cal and low-fat diets are based on packaged and processed foods that zap fat and calories from what were once whole foods, while also robbing them of nutrition and taste. In other words, they leave you unfulfilled—and desperately hungry. Not the kapha diet. Your diet features fresh and dried fruits, grains, leafy green veggies, poultry, and fish. All of these foods are light, tasty, and easily digested.

Take a look at how some of the features of the kapha diet are going to help you slim down and achieve balance.

Kapha imbalance: Slow metabolism
The fix: Slimming down with spices

The kapha diet encourages you to cook with spices. According to Ayurveda, spices stoke your digestive fire. In plain English, that means they speed up your metabolism. One study found that capsaicin, the compound that gives red chili pepper its kick, may cause the body to burn as many as 23 percent more calories. And, a breakthrough study in animals recently published in the *Journal of Nutrition* found that curcumin, the compound that gives the spice turmeric (kapha-diet approved!) its yellow hue, may halt the growth of new fat cells. Scientists believe the substance may slow the formation of new blood vessels within fat tissue, which cuts off food and oxygen required for producing new cells. Other studies have found that adding spices such as cinnamon and black pepper cause people to consume fewer calories during their meal.

Kapha Superfoods

Dried fruit

Dried fruit helps kaphas get rid of excess mucus.

Sprouts

They're rich in antioxidants and sometimes carry as much as 400 times the nutritional properties of an adult plant. They are also extremely detoxifying to the digestive system.

Bell peppers

Astringent and cooling, bell peppers are rich in vitamins A, B, and C. They naturally remove congestion and detox the blood and lymph.

Corn

This is one of the driest grains and helps combat kapha's tendency to hold on to excess mucus.

Swiss chard

A wonderful leafy green vegetable, Swiss chard cleanses the blood and lymph while providing chlorophyll to nourish the good bacteria in the gut.

Spinach

Another purifying leafy green that is rich in vitamins and minerals.

Onions

They're spicy, pungent, and astringent; as a result, they stimulate the nervous and immune systems to rejuvenate and decongest the body.

Honey

Honey is a warm, sweet, and slightly pungent sweetener that is known to aid fat burning.

Hot peppers

Spices, including peppers, boost metabolism—perfect for kapha types.

Peas

This highly nourishing spring legume is a great lymph-moving and rejuvenating food for a kapha type.

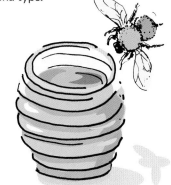

Kapha imbalance: Congestion

The fix: Nixing dairy

One big kapha diet "don't" is dairy. Dairy products are believed to increase mucus (think about drinking milk when you have a head cold), a major problem for kapha, because of a certain protein called casein. Casein may thicken existing mucus and cause a runny nose or postnasal drip. Given that you are already susceptible to congestion, you want to avoid foods that allow it to build up and exacerbate conditions such as allergies, asthma, and bronchitis. Instead, choose dairy substitutes such as soy milk or rice milk (and products made from them), which provide calcium without adding to any of the heavy, moist qualities you're trying to expel. If you find you're falling short of the recommended daily 1,000 milligrams of calcium (more if you're pregnant, nursing, or postmenopausal), we suggest taking calcium supplements that contain vitamin D to aid with absorption. And get your vitamin D_3 checked by a medical practitioner. A recent study from the *American Journal of Clinical Nutrition* estimated that 87 percent of Americans are deficient in vitamin D in the winter, and low levels of vitamin D are linked to chronic weight gain and obesity.

THE KAPHA DIET GUIDELINES

- Choose foods that are light, dry, and warm, such as leafy green veggies, berries, and grains; avoid those that are heavy and oily, such as nuts, oils, and red meat.

- Cook with more spices.

- Avoid dairy.

THE KAPHA SHOPPING LIST

The kapha body wants to cling to moisture and fat when it's out of balance. With the foods listed on the opposite page, you're going to end that once and for all. Yes, the recipes in the diet emphasize foods low in calories and fat, but you won't have to become a slave to a calculator and a food journal, tallying every morsel that passes through your lips. All of the kapha diet foods are naturally low in fat and calories because they come from the earth, not a factory. Moreover, the meal plans combine these foods in specific ways to provide the appropriate amounts of nutrients you need in each meal. Copy and post this list on your refrigerator, or leave it in your car so you always have it on hand.

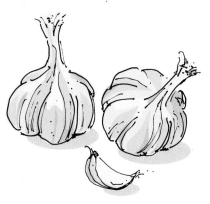

*Favor these Foods

VEGETABLES
Alfalfa sprouts*
Artichokes
Asparagus*
Bean sprouts*
Beets
Bell peppers*
Bitter melon*
Broccoli
Brussels sprouts*
Cabbage*
Carrots*
Cauliflower*
Celery*
Chicory*
Chilies, dried*
Collard greens*
Corn*
Dandelion*
Endive*
Fennel
Garlic*
Ginger
Green beans*
Hot peppers*
Jicama
Kale*
Leeks
Lettuce*
Mushrooms*
Mustard greens*
Onions*
Potatoes, baked*
Radishes*
Seaweed
Spinach*
Swiss chard*
Turnips*
Watercress*

FRUITS
All berries
Apples
Blueberries
Dried fruit (all)*
Grapefruit
Lemons
Limes
Papayas
Pears
Pomegranates
Raspberries
Strawberries

SPICES AND HERBS
Anise
Asafetida
Basil
Bay leaf
Black pepper*
Chamomile
Caraway
Cardamom
Cayenne*
Cilantro
Cinnamon
Clove*
Coriander
Cumin
Dill
Fennel
Fenugreek
Garlic
Ginger
Horseradish
Marjoram
Mustard
Nutmeg

Oregano
Parsley*
Peppermint
Poppy seeds
Rosemary
Saffron
Sage
Spearmint
Thyme
Turmeric

LEGUMES
Adzuki
All sprouted beans*
Black gram
Fava
Garbanzo
Kidney*
Lentils*
Lima*
Mung*
Peas*
Snow peas
Soy*
Split peas

MEATS AND FISH
Chicken
Freshwater fish

OILS
Canola
Corn*
Mustard
Safflower
Soy
Sunflower

DAIRY AND DAIRY SUBSTITUTES
Ghee (in moderation)
Goat milk—low-fat*
Rice milk
Soy milk

GRAINS
Amaranth
Barley
Brown rice
Buckwheat
Corn
Long grain rice
Oats
Quinoa
Rye

BEVERAGES
Water (room temperature or hot)

HERBAL TEA
Alfalfa
Cardamom*
Chicory*
Cinnamon*
Clove*
Dandelion*
Ginger*
Hibiscus*
Orange peel*
Strawberry leaf*

SWEETENERS
Honey—raw*
Molasses

De-Stress Your Diet

This plan was designed with you in mind; and as you've already seen, we mean it. From the specific food lists to the yoga postures, each step is created to balance your dosha, inspire weight loss, free your mind, and help you feel fantastic. However, we are also asking you to make some big lifestyle changes (stop snacking, for instance). Although we wish these changes could be simple and seamless for everyone, that is not the case. Over the next 3 weeks, these De-Stress Your Diet sidebars will address common problems you might experience with the week's practice and simple Zen solutions to keep you on track.

VATA

Stress: "Just the thought of only three meals a day is making me anxious."

Solution: As natural grazers, vatas may be eating as many as seven, eight, or nine times per day already, so cutting back to three is a lot to ask. Go slowly. Begin by eating breakfast, lunch, and dinner and adding a fourth meal, such as a bowl of soup, before bedtime. Listen to your body, and remember to make each meal large and satisfying, eat in a quiet setting, and go slowly.

PITTA

Stress: "I don't have time to do this."

Solution: It's true that eating three meals per day is going to require more time than you're used to, in that you typically grab food on the go and inhale it—not able to recall 5 minutes later what (or if) you just ate. Think about it like this: You wouldn't keep filling your Prius with just enough to drive to the next gas station. But that's what you're doing right now. Planning each meal—deciding before the day starts what you're going to eat and making that food readily accessible when you need it—will allow you to attack your day full-force, as you are prone to do. The payoff is that you'll be able to go through your day at 90 miles per hour without encountering a single bump in the road.

KAPHA

Stress: "I'm crashing between meals."

Solution: Kaphas will find adjusting to eating three daily meals easier than vatas or pittas. However, because you may be used to snacking, you probably have unstable blood sugar levels that cause you to crash if you go more than a few hours without eating. Fortunately, this will resolve quickly. Approach this week with the intention of eating three daily meals. However, if you feel you can't make it from one meal to the next without fading, eat a small, healthy snack.

3. Do Yoga for Your Dosha

Now that you know all about how to eat for your type, it is time to unroll your sticky mat and make your way into Downward-Facing Dog. Maybe it will be your first; maybe it will be your millionth. Either way, it will serve you. Just this simple posture releases your hips, hamstrings, and calves. It stretches your wrists, neck, and shoulders while toning your abs, arms, and back. And that's just one pose! Imagine what an entire practice can do. You're about to find out.

Just as each dosha has different nutritional requirements in order to achieve balance, each also benefits from different kinds of yoga practices. For instance, a pitta needs a slow-flowing practice to temper her fire. A vata's practice should foster inner and outer strength, while yoga for a kapha should be fast-paced and sweaty.

In the next three sections (one for each dosha), you're going to find more about why the yoga we've designed for your dosha is going to help you slim down and tone up while increasing flexibility and cultivating the clear, sharp yoga mind we introduced you to in the first chapter. You will also find a list of 20 power poses for your dosha. These are the absolute best postures—out of thousands—for you.

A Vata Yoga Practice

Even more important than the style of yoga or what poses you practice, a vata type needs postures that keep you grounded. Because you're prone to distraction and to starting projects and leaving them undone, vata workouts encourage you to drop anchor, creating physical and mental stability and strength.

Once you're on the mat, consider yourself on retreat. Ban anything in your environment that is erratic (TV blaring in the background) so that you can tune in to yourself and tune out the world. And as soon as you find the wherewithal to get through the sessions, you should congratulate yourself. The hard work will be over.

Because a vata body is usually small-framed and willowy, and because maybe for a while you got away with being skinny but not strong, you may find the muscle-building poses uncomfortable at first. If your legs shimmy and shake, don't worry. Tremors and wobbles mean that your skeleton is being tested, and you are building bone mass and retraining your muscles to keep you steady. Despite their light and feathery look, vatas usually have extraordinary strength. If you have some flab you want the yoga to devour, use the demanding poses to draw the muscle to the bone and extend your limbs for a few extra inches. Even perking up your posture can give you the look of a few pounds lost.

If you are looking for classes in your area, aim for a class that trains you for advanced poses and emphasizes breathing. The key words you should look for are hatha, vinyasa, or flow. These types of classes offer a buffet of the regular yoga fare: standing, forward bending, back bending, twisting, and inverted postures. Your body needs equal amounts of stretching and sculpting, which these classes offer, and your mind will like the variety. You want to avoid classes that emphasize only one facet of yoga such as those labeled *restorative* or *yin*. (Don't get us wrong: We love all yoga, but you're looking for what's going to have the biggest payoffs over the next 3 weeks. We encourage you to work toward trying all varieties of yoga when you have achieved the desired results from this plan.)

If any of this is anxiety provoking, take a step back and come back to simple breaths. Your creative mind will surely lead you to stretches that your body needs for some serious sculpting. Respect it.

20 Power Poses for Vatas*

These are the absolute best poses for vatas. When these come up in yoga class or you have a few extra minutes at home pay special attention to these postures. (Don't get distracted; you can stick to this plan). Try to stay focused on how they feel. You want to approach the practice steadily, finding a balance between building strength and letting go. Some of these poses will address your body's automatic response to long holds—it will want to move on in favor of snappier moves. But if you find yourself wishing you could move on, hurry a bit, or try something new, encourage yourself to find the inner discipline to hold the pose for just one more breath. This will allow you to go a little deeper into the pose than you have before. That novelty should keep you engaged.

How to Use this List at Home

The practice will take approximately 20 to 30 minutes. Always start with 10 Sun Salutations. (See the Sun Salutation illustration on page 224.) The first one should be slow and breathy. Take a minimum of one full, complete breath (inhale and exhale) in each posture of your Sun Salutation. Worry less about the form and more about opening up the noticeably tight spots in your body. On the fifth Sun Salutation, be a bit more exact about your form. Begin matching one movement (Upward-Facing Dog to Downward-Facing Dog, for example) with one inhalation or exhalation. Make your last four Sun Salutes faster, and hit each position like a gymnast.

Mentally, vatas have a tough time getting focused. If setting a mental intention works for you, use it. In a position on your mat, cross your nondominant ankle in front of you and place your right palm face up inside the left upward facing palm. Breathe naturally and make a wish. Yoga teachers call these "intentions," but just a single thought, from "patience" to "cook a healthy dinner tonight," is a powerful way to rein in a busy mind. If your mind wanders as the yoga moves unravel, revisit the thought. Or if you have a pose you are holding, you can repeat the word or phrase until it becomes white noise.

After your mind and body warm up and you feel calmer and your muscles let go of some tension, choose five of the moves listed here. Do each move for at least 5 to 10 breaths. The longer you hold the position, the more stress you bust and flab you tighten. If you find yourself tensing up or holding your breath, take Child's Pose and then revisit the position. If you can hold the move and keep your breath steady for 5-to-10 full, complete breaths, you are reaping the intended benefits.

Why did we select these as the best poses for airy types? They all encourage three projects critical for vata types to build a balanced, grounded routine despite the distractions around them: building total body strength, creating greater stability, and balancing the mind and the body equally.

1. Plank: Recruits the core muscles, develops emotional strength, and enhances confidence

2. Downward-Facing Dog: Energizes; opens arms, shoulders, back, and legs

3. Upward-Facing Dog: Opens the chest while strengthening the back; improves mood and combats depression and anxiety

4. Forward Fold: Releases the back and tailbone; opens the backs of legs and hip joints while encouraging introspection

5. Low Pushup: Strengthens the total body; shapes the arms, and builds the chest, back, and core muscles

6. Dolphin: Encourages circulation, builds upper body and core strength, prepares the body for head and hand stands

7. Warrior I: Combats stress, insomnia, and anxiety; encourages balance and builds strength

8. Triangle: Stretches the side body, allowing the legs to ground down and release low spine tension while the spine gets longer

9. Warrior III: Requires balance and total body strength. Builds balance.

10. Revolved Half-Moon: Encourages better digestion, and as a fusion of twist and balance, makes one stronger, longer, and a more effective multitasker

11. Eagle: Squeezes tension out of the hips, back, and shoulders, allowing the core to be the main source of strength

12. Dancer: Combines balance with strength. Requires the spine and back to release tension

13. Tree: Fosters focus, ignite the core, and encourages balance

14. Crow: Requires deep core strength, overcoming fear of falling forward

15. Frog: Unleashes toxic emotions believed to be stored in fatty tissue, especially the hips; frees up the spine and tailbone; lubricates creaky joints, especially in the hips

16. Plow: Stretches the neck and spine, encouraging the nervous system to relax

17. One-Legged Downward-Facing Dog: Adds a strengthening element to a restful total-body toning pose

18. Side Plank with Single Toe Hold: Allows the body to work dynamically, toning the inner legs, core, and arms while tightening the tummy

19. Half-Moon with Bent Knee: Requires focused attention to balance, combined with the strength of being on one leg; invites a backbend to increase openness in the front body

20. Alternate Nostril Breathing: Balances right and left brain; encourages creativity

*Find all of these poses illustrated in Chapter 9. Instructions for Alternative Nostril Breathing are on page 93.

A Pitta Yoga Practice

The primary goal of a pitta-balancing yoga practice is to leave the competitive streak at home. Ultimately, your ability to be the best won't win you any points in yoga. For you, triumph is assuming Child's Pose instead of squeezing out another Sun Salutation at your joints' expense. Pittas excel where goals are obvious and challenges can be overcome. Rather than pretending you don't care about goals, reset them. Rather than being the most flexible or strongest yogini in the room, be competitive and aggressive about how much you can hold back or how carefully you can execute a slow, precise flow series. Slow motion for you will bring your awareness to your body and flavor your practice with an energy that will endure rather than exhaust.

A pitta's life is full of fire; but on the yoga mat, you want to take your boiling point down to a simmer. The real work for pittas is to do less and to feel good about it. When a teacher offers an advanced pose, try not to take the plunge unless you've maxed out at the prior level. Commit to the current sensations and then go deeper. If this approach dulls the thrill, then go ahead and jump; but do it the way a dancer leaps—like taffy being pulled rather than a Teenage Mutant Ninja Turtle hurling sloppily through space.

When practicing yoga, pitta types should home in on the forward folds and the seated poses. Forward folds encourage introspection; they help you look inside yourself and ask what is going on and what you really want. (Plus, you won't be comparing yourself to the girl on the mat next to you.) Reducing the stimuli allows the nervous system to relax. And when you're in long, deep, seated poses, your intensity will be met with your body's heightened sensations of deep-tissues release.

As the sensations intensify, see if you can use your breath—slow, deep inhalations and exhalations in and out of the nose—to stay longer and quieter in the pose. The more a pitta's mind and body give in, the more she'll get from the pose. Plus, this approach sends stress packing. Only a pitta has the ability to make yoga stressful! Don't do it.

If you are researching types of classes to attend locally, a restorative class at the end of the week will leave you feeling as rested as you'd feel if you'd slept for a decade. This type of active rest is just what you need to accomplish even more than you already do. Another option is to try yoga styles such as Iyengar or Anusara. These techniques emphasize alignment, which will help balance your goal-oriented mind. Instead of trying to out-yoga your classmates or do the very best Upward-Facing Dog the world has ever witnessed, you will shift your focus to making sure your bellybutton is pulling toward your spine and your shoulder blades are pressing down your back in every pose.

If you come to understand the finer points of the mind-body exercise—such as how to use the inner thighs and big toes for stability or how to use your third eye for creativity—you'll add a mental challenge to the practice allowing you to escape your to-do list and tune in to the dynamic movements required to attune your body to the detail it takes to achieve head-to-toe health.

Remember, every yoga pose is good for you, but your "power poses" will encourage you to work toward a different kind of perfection: the kind that's perfectly accepting of the imperfect.

20 Power Poses for Pittas*

When these come up in yoga class or you have a few extra minutes at home (you're a pitta—you can find the time to wedge it in between work and play) take a special interest in how you perform them and whether they make you feel more present and available. They should. Use these poses when you start panicking about your racing pulse. Or if you sense you need some extra ammunition against oncoming stress, step onto the mat or carpet and try some prescription yoga. While you could thrive in a speedy vinyasa flow class or look impressive keeping up with the hot yoga team, your challenge is to slow down your practice in order to build strength and agility.

How to Use this List at Home

Usually, a cool-down ends a class, but pitta people need to begin with one. The best recommendation is to begin on your back. Lie on your back, close your eyes, draw the soles of your feet together, and place your hand on your belly. Let your whole body go slack and just watch your breath. Stay this way while you count 10 breaths. Then roll onto your right side and use your palms to come to a seated position. Cross your nondominant ankle in front of you and place your right palm face up, inside the left upward-facing palm. Breathe naturally and make a wish. Yoga teachers call these "intentions," but a just single thought, from "patience" to "cook a healthy dinner tonight," is a powerful way to rein in a busy mind. If your mind wanders as the yoga moves unravel, revisit the thought. Or if you have a pose you are holding, you can repeat this word or phrase until it becomes white noise.

After your mind and body warm up and calm sets in, choose five of the moves listed here. Do each move for at least 5 to 10 breaths. The longer you hold the position, the more stress you bust and flab you tighten. If you find yourself tensing up or holding your breath, take Child's Pose and then revisit the position. If you can hold the move and keep your breath steady for 5 to 10 full, complete breaths, you are reaping the intended benefits.

The practice will take approximately 20 to 30 minutes. Always start with 10 Sun Salutations. (See the Sun Salutation illustration on page 224.) The first one should be slow and breathy. Take a minimum of one full, complete breath (inhale and exhale) in each posture making up your Sun Salutation. Worry less about the form and more about opening up the noticeably tight spots in your body. On the fifth Sun Salutation, be a bit more exact about your form. Begin matching one movement (Upward-Facing Dog to Downward-Facing Dog, for example) with one inhalation or exhalation. Make your last four Sun Salutes faster, and hit each position like a gymnast. The faster you move, the more in control of your body you appear.

An antidote to fiery pitta tendencies is to choose poses that encourage calm intensity, which is a pitta's trump card. Deep, long holds can untangle years of tucked away tension. Perfect poses for pitta include those that require the body to let go and release rather than heat and fire muscles; strength-building poses that challenge you to create a deep mind-body connection to achieve intricate shapes; and poses that require long holds by squeezing, twisting, or folding in order to release trapped muscle tissue.

1. Downward-Facing Dog: Serves as a cool-down during fast flows; an inversion, it offers calm and total body lengthening

2. Warrior II: Enables the hips to open and the spine to release stored tension

3. Revolved Triangle: Opens and stretches the legs, hips, and side body while adding a twist to encourage better digestion

4. Tree with Lotus: Improves strength in the ankles and legs while opening the hips and requiring balance

5. Crow: Requires deep core strength; teaches the body to let go in some muscle groups and to engage others in a dynamic balance

6. Double Toe Hold: Requires an extreme lengthening of the spine and legs

7. Locust: Strengthens and tones the back of the body

8. Camel: Improves the mood and opens the front body, shoulders, and upper back

9. Bridge with Roll: Lifts the mood as a backbend does, but the added leg activity encourages core strength and mental focus

10. Supported Fish: Opens the chest, improves the mood, supports the spine, and opens the hips

11. Reclined Cobbler: Releases the inner groin and legs while allowing the spine to de-stress

12. Cow Face: Removes cellulite by increasing lymph flow

13. Frog: Unleashes toxic emotions believed to be stored in fatty tissue, especially hips; frees up the spine and tailbone; lubricates creaky joints, especially those in the hips

14. Plow: Stretches the neck and spine, encouraging the nervous system to relax

15. Happy Baby: Opens hips. Promotes relaxation.

16. Double Pigeon: Squeezes tension out of the deep hips; encourages calm, release, and introspection

17. Hero: Fights fatigue; fires up circulation in the legs and spine

18. Legs Up the Wall: Allows swelling and inflammation in the legs to subside while releasing the spine

19. Bow: A backbend that encourages shoulder opening and total body expansion.

20. Alternate Nostril Breathing: Balances right and left brain; encourages creativity

*Find all of these poses illustrated in Chapter 9. Instructions for Alternate Nostril Breathing are on page 93.

A KAPHA YOGA PRACTICE

A kapha practice is hotter and sweatier than that of any other type. The primary goals for kaphas are to get working and to break out of routine in order to slim down bulky muscles and make fat melt off. The best yoga for you will create heat (called *tapas* in Sanskrit) in the body and burn off the toxins you've tucked away. By aggressively building heat, increasing heart rate, and stoking your mental fires, your yoga practice can break up the body's congestion.

Where kaphas—in life—may tend toward an elegant routine and organized system of planning and executing, on the yoga mat they need to be a force of nature. If you've done 3 years of kickboxing but you still don't have the muscle definition you want, this routine and the reasons why you need it will have some serious resonance. If you've worked out without results, you may have continued to exercise only the parts of the body that you are conditioned to recruit. In yoga, you want to use variety and spontaneity. Counter to your customary, ingrained way of working out, your yoga practice will be quick and dynamic. Every minute should encourage you to let go and flow.

Kaphas should favor creative hybrids, vinyasa, fusions (yoga on the ball, yogalates), and fast-flow classes. You are also a good candidate for hot yoga (sometimes called Bikram) because the external heat will encourage you to heat up internally, which can decrease bloating and get you moving. Sessions where you move quickly through poses, encounter a bit of the unexpected in pose choreography, and also feel your heart rate soar are good for burning fat, decreasing cellulite, and making the mental adjustment to not fall back on habit.

Which poses accomplish weight loss and muscle toning for kaphas? Most of the poses in your list of 20 power poses target large muscle groups such as the legs and glutes. As for your practice, favor fun. Don't be shy. Throw your weight around. Jumping from pose to pose and attacking the pose will increase the cardio factor and help you burn fat faster.

Remember, every yoga pose is good for you, but your "power poses" take you out of your comfort zone and expressly recruit the larger muscles in your body to burn fat faster.

20 POWER POSES FOR KAPHAS*

When these come up in yoga class or you have a few extra minutes at home (we know—who are we kidding?), that's a sign for you to go for it. These poses are your quick fixes. Better than forward folds that encourage introspection and slowing down the bodily system, these are big and athletic. Kapha yoga challenges the body to

work so hard it can't help burning fat and building muscle.

How to Use this List at Home

The practice will take approximately 20 to 30 minutes. Always start with 10 Sun Salutations. (See the Sun Salutation illustration on page 224.) The first one should be slow and breathy. Take a minimum of one full, complete breath (inhale and exhale) in each posture making up your Sun Salutation. Worry less about the form and more about opening up the noticeably tight spots in your body. On the fifth Sun Salutation, be a bit more exact about your form. Begin matching one movement (Upward-Facing Dog to Downward-Facing Dog, for example) with one inhalation or exhalation. Make your last four Sun Salutes faster, and hit each position like a gymnast. The faster you move, the more in control of your body you appear.

Earth types crawl onto their mats, but they need a little more mojo. Try to take the routine out of your practice not by varying the time and place, necessarily, but by asking a bit more of yourself. Stay on that mat for 10 more minutes if you can; muscle out a few more of the poses; push yourself. You'll be happy to find yourself taking wider stances. Making your moves bigger isn't embarrassing, it's empowering. It's good for a grounded kapha to begin with a spicy intention. In yoga-speak, the "intention" is like making a wish.

To begin, sit on the floor and cross your nondominant ankle in front of you and place your right palm face up, inside the left upward-facing palm. Breathe naturally and make a wish. This "intention," which may be just a single thought, from "patience" to "cook a healthy dinner tonight," is a powerful way to rein in a busy mind. If your mind wanders as the yoga moves unravel, revisit the thought. Or if you have a pose you are holding, you can repeat this word or phrase until it becomes white noise.

After your mind and body warm up and you feel calmer and your muscles let go of some tension, choose five of the moves listed here. Do each move for at least 5 to 10 breaths. The longer you hold the position, the more stress you bust and flab you tighten. If you find yourself tensing up or holding your breath, take Child's Pose and then revisit the position. If you can hold the move and keep your breath steady for 5 to 10 full, complete breaths, you are reaping the intended benefits.

Why did we select these as the best poses for kaphas? They all encourage three projects that both on and off the mat are critical for earth types: to build strength, break out of a rut, and increase metabolism.

1. Sun Salutation: Energizes, tones, and conditions the total body; relaxes the nervous system

2. Plank: Recruits core muscles, develops emotional strength, and enhances confidence

3. Cobra: Improves mood; opens and strengthens the chest; strengthens the back and shoulders

4. Upward-Facing Dog: Opens the chest while strengthening the back; improves the mood and combats depression and anxiety

5. Low Pushup: Increases confidence, builds core and arm strength, and lengthens the legs

6. Dolphin: Encourages circulation, builds upper body and core strength, prepares the body for head and hand stands

7. Chair: Strengthens the total body

8. Dancer: Recruits total body strength and balance; tones legs, back, and core while opening chest and giving spine length and strength.

9. Warrior III: Requires a strong core to stand on one leg; recruits the back muscles

10. Reverse Warrior: Opens the front body (groin, legs, chest); empowers while grounding; fights fatigue

11. Crow: Requires deep core strength; teaches the body to let go in some muscle groups and engage others in a dynamic balance

12. Boat: Requires balance, leg strength, and a strong core

13. Bow: Stimulates endocrine, digestive, and respiratory systems while massaging abdomen and spine

14. Shoulder Stand: Relaxes the nervous system; stretches the spine and tailbone; builds confidence; improves mental acuity

15. Reverse Plank: Opens the chest; stretches the front of the body from head to toe; works the arms, glutes, and core

16. L-Seat: Improves concentration; increases strength in the arms, core, and legs

17. Rock 'n' Roll Pushup: Requires total body control and extra strength in the abs

18. One-Legged Downward-Facing Dog: Adds a strengthening element to a restful total-body toning pose

19. Lunge with Power Forward Arms: Strengthens core; creates fire in the abdomen; recruits the big muscle groups to burn fat

20. Alternate Nostril Breathing: Balances right and left brain; encourages creativity

*Find all of these poses in Chapter 9. Instructions for Alternate Nostril Breathing are on page 93.

5

WEEK 3: HEALTHY HABITS TO BURN FAT FASTER

Dismiss whatever insults your own soul.
—*Walt Whitman*

In 2 weeks' time, you've taught your body to burn fat again. You've taken the stress down a notch with simple techniques like calm mealtimes and yoga for your type. You should be burning fat again and fighting stress better. By now, you should be feeling naturally cleaner, healthier, and lighter.

Think of the first 2 weeks as preparation for the last two. In other words, you've set yourself up to become a fat-burning machine, and now you're going to ask the body to do even more—

because it's ready. Going to three meals a day and staying hydrated most likely eliminated your cravings and improved your digestion. Now it's time to make your blood sugar as reliable as Air Force One. Adding one simple mealtime technique to the program will send your body into super fat-burn mode. Specifically, we're going to help you optimize your health and encourage daily weight loss (or ideal weight maintenance) by ensuring that your blood sugar stays steady.

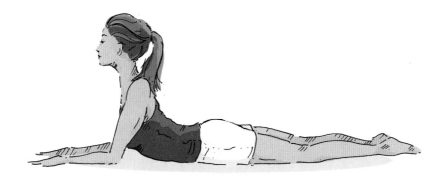

The Blood Sugar Connection

When you eat, food gets converted into glucose, your body's and brain's favorite fuel. However, if you eat a meal with too much starch or too much sugar, your body receives more glucose than it needs. So, the body releases insulin, a hormone produced by the pancreas to bring blood sugar levels back down. Insulin directs the sugar into cells and stores it in muscles. At moderate levels, this process is fairly stable. However, if you eat several slices of pizza, a plate of fries, or a mountain of mashed potatoes, your body has to deal with a tsunami of blood sugar.

What does it do? It floods the body with *more* insulin to drive blood sugar levels down. The problem is, the pancreas pumps out so much insulin that blood sugar levels plummet. In fact, your blood sugar can drop even lower than it was before you ate. So even though you may have consumed enough calories for two meals, before long, your body receives the signal that it is starved, and the brain sends out hunger cues.

Hello, cravings! You're sent foraging for food despite the fact that you're still contending with sugar overload. Your body is in a constant state of panic. The mind-body chaos makes us feel spent and low. As the effects of spikes and crashes in blood sugar, we struggle with hunger confusion, cravings met and unmet, fatigue, and mania.

The other thing that occurs when your pancreas is pouring out insulin is that the body ceases to burn fat so it can run on glucose instead. This makes losing weight virtually impossible.

Take a deep breath. Now that you know what's going on, you can ground yourself by choosing a food fix for your type, which will make you feel stable, energized, and mentally clear. Cutting out snacks was your first line of defense.

These next 2 weeks are going to continue remedying blood sugar instability by keeping levels on a more even keel, with a special emphasis on sending the body into fat-burning mode for longer periods. There's no need to starve or fast. A good night's sleep is about as close to fasting as you'll get. If you follow the next steps, you'll "fast" all night, every night, as nature intended. The result? More time burning fat. And your body burns fat faster because it's not busy with (1) the blood sugar tsunami, and (2) digestive processes that compete for your body's energy while you are asleep. According to Ayurveda, the "janitor" comes at night and cleans up your insides so you'll look great outside. If he can't do his work because the night school's in session, then you won't be thoroughly prepared for the next day.

Here are the simple keys to burning fat faster and longer, as well as guidelines for making them part of your life despite a long list of daily demands. We offer these steps at the midpoint of this plan because you're ready. Your body is ready.

1. Eat Lunch; Shrink Dinner

This week you're going to make lunch the biggest meal of your day. Why? Ayurveda says that your metabolism and digestive strength peak between 10:00 a.m. and 2:00 p.m. Therefore, you should max out on calories at lunch, when your body will digest the meal most efficiently. Plus, these days noon is the new 9:00 a.m. We are just getting started on our day and topping off that coffee, even if we've risen at 5:00 a.m. When the clock strikes noon, you still have a full day ahead of you. Eat for it.

Of course, we live in a society where the lunch hour has gone the way of snail mail (clunky, slow, and easily avoidable), but let's try to recall the practice of eating in peace. *The Yoga Body Diet* takes into account that you are not frequently going to be able to sit down to a large, sedate meal in the middle of your day. We know that you don't have someone cooking for you all day.

But we encourage you to try eating a bigger lunch and smaller dinner at least three times this week and to work that habit into your weekend. You will feel the results. Notice what happens around the time that you usually experience a slump (for most of us, it's around 3:00 or 4:00 p.m.). Those 20 minutes you took to enjoy a hearty meal will send you breezing through the afternoon without a hitch. Relying on granola fumes, on the other hand, may mean that only an intravenous drip of espresso will get you through to dinnertime.

We like to think that the word "supper" actually means that that meal is "supplemental." Lunch is where the main action occurs.

The Week 3 Meal Plan

This plan refers to the recipes in Chapter 8.

Choose any breakfast from the recipes starting on page 96.

• For lunch, choose any lunch or dinner recipe. Eat dessert with your midday meal, too. Depending on your individual activity and hunger levels, if you think you need more food at this meal, increase the quantity, add a side of soup, or make extra veggies from your list. If it looks like a lot of food, that's because it is—and that is okay.

• For dinner, have either a soup or a salad. If you are a vata, you should always choose soup, because it is warm and moist. Pittas and kaphas can have either.

2. Do Yoga For Your Dosha

People often talk about how their body was reshaped after they took up yoga. It's true. The total body conditioning that yoga offers, paired with the ease with which you can practice, makes it a simple, accessible, and effective.

You've eased into a practice with simple breathing techniques; and hopefully, after test-driving the 20 Power Poses for your type, you've found a half-dozen poses that de-stress your body. But now it's time to make yoga a workout. We've put together three classes for each dosha, themed to accomplish the common goals for that type. Where core strength was paramount for a wobbly vata, we prescribe a class that combats a weak and wiggly center. For fiery pitta types, who need to calm some of their restlessness, there are sequences that make them sit and stay. And for grounded, ritualized kaphas, there are three classes that will push them to move out of their comfort zones and fire up their metabolism.

How do you use these workouts? Each of the three workouts for your type runs 30, 60, or 90 minutes. We suggest you practice three times a week. In a perfect world, you would do the 30-minute sequence one day, the 60-minute sequence the next day, and then the 90-minute sequence the next. But in real life, if you manage

De-Stress Your Diet

VATA

Stress: "I still want a big dinner."

Solution: You might not be ready to shrink dinner yet, and that's okay. You took the biggest step by going from too many meals to count, to three or four. This week, focus on getting rid of the fourth meal and eating three big ones. By now your blood sugar is stable enough to get you happily from meal to meal without severe hunger or sluggishness. If you aren't satisfied, choose a snack of fruit or nuts.

PITTA

Stress: "Why should I bother with supper anyway, if we're making it so small? I can skip it."

Solution: Pitta's efficiency makes her want to skip anything extra. But it's not overkill to eat three times a day; it's essential. Although skipping supper is an option next week (You peeked, didn't you?), this week, stick to three meals, making lunch bigger and dinner smaller. Ditching supper now will communicate to your nervous system that you're under duress, and it will likely respond with stress and anxiety. Stay calm and present, and steady your eating habits. Even though we know you're tough enough to go for it, take the easy way out this time. Trust us.

KAPHA

Stress: "These meals are too light. I miss my cream and cheese!"

Solution: Kaphas love their heavy comfort foods, especially those made with creams and cheese. However, dairy products are responsible for many of kapha's weight-gaining tendencies, which are related to excess mucus production. Here's what to do if you get hit by cravings or you feel that a meal (especially dinner this week) isn't satisfying enough: Increase the quantity. Eat two bowls of soup, if you need to. Redefine for yourself what "satisfied" means. It doesn't have to be ice cream at 10:00 p.m. with the TV on. If you find a salad leaves you hungry, add lean protein, to it, such as grilled chicken, fish, or tofu. You'll know you're satisfied when the cravings subside. Try hot water and add a tablespoon of honey. Honey has fat-burning properties.

to get in three good sessions during a week, God bless.

You can also use the sequences for half of the time prescribed by holding each pose half the time recommended. That will give you 15-minute, 30-minute, and 45-minute sequences based on the longer versions.

Be creative; allow yourself to try different things. If you get stuck in one pose, go with it. And if you want to cross over and borrow a core sequence from vata even though you're a die-hard kapha, do it. Any yoga will encourage weight loss, stress reduction, and a lean physique. We've offered sequences to optimize balance in your type, but we welcome you to try what appeals to you and keep what sticks. Any other philosophy would contradict the yoga principle. Your workouts should be individualized. You know what your body needs better than anyone else.

VATA'S YOGA WORKOUTS

It is critical for vatas to be able to stand tall and strong. Balancing poses are good for you. If you can rein in the wavering and waffling of the body and mind while you are standing on one leg as secure as Lady Liberty, you can take some of that added stability off the mat with you. Standing poses recruit the core and cause you to strengthen your legs. You may notice that by plugging your big toe into the floor, you are required to recruit the inner leg muscles—so your hard-to-reach inner thighs will become less jiggly. As for your yoga butt, these sequences are designed to firm the derriere. No matter what flurry of activity begs for your attention, these poses will help you keep the mind from wandering and the waist from growing so much as an inch.

Continue to do the breathing technique (that you learned on page 21) five days a week for 10 minutes a day.

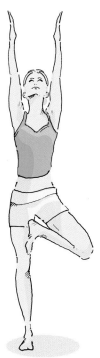

Vata's yoga workout schedule looks like this:

Workout 1: 30-Minute Fat-Blasting Balancing Sequence
Workout 2: 60-Minute Grounding Sequence
Workout 3: 90 Minutes of Total Body Conditioning
(Go to www.theyogabodydiet.com to download music playlists for these workouts.)

30-Minute Fat-Blasting Balancing Sequence (Vata)

POSE NAME	BREATHS (FULL INHALATION AND EXHALATION)	REPS
Cow/Cat	4	4
Cow/Cat Pointer (each side)	4	4
Forward Fold	5	1
Sun Salutation A	9	1
Upward-Facing Dog	8	1
Downward-Facing Dog	8	1
Low Pushup	4	1
Downward-Facing Dog	8	1
Low Pushup	4	1
Sun Salutation B	9	1
Warrior I (each side)	8	1
Forward Fold	8	1
Tree (left leg)	5	1
Tree with Lotus (left leg)	5	1
Tree (right leg)	5	1
Tree with Lotus (right leg)	5	1
Eagle (each side)	10	1
Dancer (each leg)	10	1
Pigeon (each side)	10	1
Double Pigeon (each side)	10	1
Frog	10	1
Reclined Twist (each side)	8	1
Corpse	10	1
TOTAL TIME: 30 MINUTES		

60-Minute Grounding Sequence (Vata)

POSE NAME	BREATHS (FULL INHALATION AND EXHALATION)	REPS
Reclined Cobbler	10	1
Cow/Cat	1	4
Sun Salutation A	4	5
Plank to Downward-Facing Dog	1	10

POSE NAME	BREATHS (FULL INHALATION AND EXHALATION)	REPS
Dolphin	5	1
Sun Salutation A	4	5
Dolphin	5	1
Sun Salutation B	5	1
Plank to Downward-Facing Dog	1	10
Dolphin	5	1
Sun Salutation B	5	1
Warrior II (right leg)	8	1
Sun Salutation B	5	1
Warrior II (left leg)	8	1
Sun Salutation B	5	1
Warrior I (right leg)	8	1
Sun Salutation B	5	1
Warrior I (left leg)	8	1
Sun Salutation B	5	1
Side Plank (each side)	8	2
Sun Salutation B	5	1
Triangle (right side)	8	1
Revolved Triangle (right side)	8	1
Sun Salutation B	5	1
Triangle (left side)	8	1
Revolved Triangle (left side)	8	1
Sun Salutation B	5	1
Tree (right side)	5	1
Tree with Lotus (right side)	5	1
Tree (left side)	5	1
Tree with Lotus (left side)	5	1
Boat	4	1
Reverse Plank	4	1
Boat	4	1
Reverse Plank	4	1
Pigeon (each leg)	10	1
Cow Face (each side)	10	1
Seated Head to Knee (each side)	10	1

(continued)

POSE NAME	BREATHS (FULL INHALATION AND EXHALATION)	REPS
Bridge	8	3
Supported Fish	10	1
Reclined Twist (each side)	10	1
Corpse	20	1

TOTAL TIME: 60 MINUTES

90 Minutes of Total Body Conditioning (Vata)

POSE NAME	BREATHS (FULL INHALATION AND EXHALATION)	REPS
Lotus	20	1
Mountain	10	1
Sun Salutation A	9	3
One-Legged Downward-Facing Dog	8	1
Sun Salutation B	9	1
Dolphin	8	1
Crow	8	2
Dolphin	8	1
Crow	8	2
Reverse Plank	8	2
Sun Salutation B	4	3
Cobra	8	2
Sun Salutation A & B	9	3
Warrior I (each side)	8	1
Warrior II (each side)	10	1
Warrior III (each side)	10	1
Forward Fold	10	1
Tree (each side)	10	1
Dancer (each side)	20	1
Sun Salutation A & B	9	3
Warrior III (right leg)	8	1
Half-Moon (right leg)	8	1
Revolved Half-Moon (right leg)	8	1
Tree (right leg)	4	1

POSE NAME	BREATHS (FULL INHALATION AND EXHALATION)	REPS
Sun Salutation A	9	3
Warrior III (left leg)	8	1
Half-Moon (left leg)	8	1
Revolved Half-Moon (left leg)	8	1
Tree (left leg)	4	1
Sun Salutation B	9	3
Locust	8	2
Sun Salutation A	4	1
Frog	10	1
Bridge	8	3
Bridge with Roll	8	3
Shoulder Stand	10	1
Plow	10	1
Reclined Twist (each side)	10	1
Corpse	25	1
TOTAL TIME: 90 MINUTES		

Pitta's Yoga Workouts

Pittas can thrive on yoga, but they have to be really careful that the practice doesn't exacerbate some of their alpha tendencies. It's best to build in 10 minutes to unwind before class starts so that you can relax before you begin. Fire types are expert at storing tension in deep tissue and walking around in the world as if they were easy and breezy. The project for a pitta is to truly unwind—to excavate the deepest recesses in her body to release built-up tension and to soften the mind. If you notice you have white knuckles or a wrinkled forehead, let go more. Don't worry about being perfect; focus more on loosening up. Being uptight and agenda-oriented always helps get the job, but during yoga you may be adding pressure to your mind and body to perform. If you can let go of the need to be perfect, you can begin to do your yoga well. If your wrists feel shaky because your practice isn't what it was last year, crawl into Child's Pose. Consider that a victory. Your mantra is "Sit, stay, *heal*." You need to stay put and find a place where you can calm down and breathe more deeply. Stop striving for perfection in a pose. Connect to your breathing, and oxygenate your body. You'll feel and look better if your endurance is focused on increasing deep release rather than accomplishing hard moves or dancing through gymnastic-like flows.

Continue to do the breathing technique (that you learned on page 21) five days a week for 10 minutes a day.

Pitta's yoga workout schedule looks like this:

Workout 1: Cool and Cut in 30 Minutes
Workout 2: Centered and Sleek in 60 Minutes
Workout 3: 90-Minute Crash Course to Chill
(Go to www.theyogabodydiet.com to download music playlists for these workouts.)

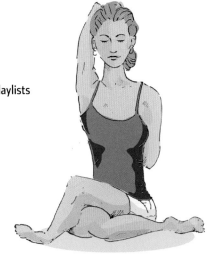

Cool and Cut in 30 Minutes (Pitta)

POSE NAME	BREATHS (FULL INHALATION AND EXHALATION)	REPS
Reclined Cobbler	10	1
Downward-Facing Dog	5	1
Plank	4	1
Low Pushup	4	1
Downward-Facing Dog	5	1
Sun Salutation A	9	2
Warrior II (left leg)	4	1
Triangle (left leg)	4	1
Half-Moon (left leg)	4	1
Sun Salutation B	9	1
Warrior II (right leg)	4	1
Triangle (right side)	4	1
Half-Moon (right leg)	4	1
Sun Salutation A	9	1
Cow Face (right leg)	8	1
Pigeon (right leg)	4	1
Double Pigeon (right leg)	8	1
Cow Face (left leg)	8	1
Pigeon (left leg)	4	1
Double Pigeon (left leg)	8	1
Camel	8	1
Supported Fish	4	1
Corpse	10	1
TOTAL TIME: 30 MINUTES		

Centered and Sleek in 60 Minutes (Pitta)

POSE NAME	BREATHS (FULL INHALATION AND EXHALATION)	REPS
Cow/Cat	1	4
Cow/Cat Pointer (each side)	1	4
Sun Salutation A	4	5
Cobra	4	1
Upward-Facing Dog	4	1
Downward-Facing Dog	4	1
Plank	4	1
Downward-Facing Dog	4	1
Cobra	8	1
Upward-Facing Dog	8	1
Downward-Facing Dog	8	1
Plank	8	1
Downward-Facing Dog	8	1
Sun Salutation A	4	2
Sun Salutation B	5	2
Pigeon (each side)	8	1
Sun Salutation A	4	2
Warrior II (each side)	5	2
Twisting Chair (each side)	8	1
Warrior II (each side)	8	1
Warrior III (right leg)	8	1
Half Moon (right leg)	8	1
Warrior III (left leg)	8	1
Half Moon (left leg)	8	1
Sun Salutation B	5	2
Side Plank (each side)	8	1
Standing Split (each side)	10	1
Squat	10	2
Camel	10	3
Pigeon (each side)	10	1
Double Pigeon (each side)	10	1
Cow Face (each side)	10	1

POSE NAME	BREATHS (FULL INHALATION AND EXHALATION)	REPS
Plow	10	1
Reclined Cobbler	10	1
Windshield Wiper (each side)	8	1
Corpse	20	1

TOTAL TIME: 60 MINUTES

90-Minute Crash Course to Chill (Pitta)

POSE NAME	BREATHS (FULL INHALATION AND EXHALATION)	REPS
Lotus	10	1
Seated Staff	5	1
Cow/Cat	4	4
Cow/Cat Pointer (each side)	4	4
Sun Salutation A	9	5
Low Pushup	4	1
Plank	4	1
Low Pushup	4	1
Plank	4	1
Low Pushup	4	1
Plank	4	1
Sun Salutation B	9	5
Warrior II (left leg)	4	1
Triangle (left leg)	4	1
Sun Salutation A	9	5
Warrior II (right leg)	4	1
Triangle (right leg)	4	1
Sun Salutation B	9	5
Warrior I (left leg)	4	1
Reverse Warrior (left leg)	4	1

(continued)

POSE NAME	BREATHS (FULL INHALATION AND EXHALATION)	REPS
Sun Salutation A	9	5
Warrior I (right leg)	4	1
Reverse Warrior (right leg)	4	1
Sun Salutation B	9	5
Lunge with Power Forward Arms (left leg)	8	1
Extended Side Angle (left leg)	8	1
Sun Salutation B	9	1
Lunge with Power Forward Arms (right leg)	8	1
Extended Side Angle (right leg)	8	1
L-Seat (each leg)	8	2
Seated Half Twist (each side)	8	1
Seated Staff	10	1
Reverse Plank	8	1
Side Plank (each side)	8	2
Pigeon (each side)	10	1
King Pigeon (each side)	10	1
Hero	5	1
Camel	5	1
Twelve Point	5	1
Reclined Cobbler	10	1
Reclined Twist (each side)	10	1
Corpse	20	1

TOTAL TIME: 90 MINUTES

Kapha's Yoga Workouts

While kaphas may feel like slinking from pose to pose, you need to strike your poses with more flair. If your metabolism is sluggish but you are peaceful in nature, you have to kick the flows up a notch.

Get comfortable being tougher from the get-go. In the past you may have worked up to the stronger, faster moves. See if you can try the harder moves early on—and enjoy it. Connect with your muscles faster. Get them firing quicker. Use your breath to keep the pacing manageable. You don't want to be beet red and panting in Downward-Facing Dog, but you should feel your heartbeat in your chest. If you don't, speed it up.

Activate your strong muscles and get them moving. If you do increase the pace and body work required, you'll notice a bit more radiance in the mirror and a sleeker body, head to toe. And you won't be so beholden to routine. Who knows; maybe it's holding you back a bit?

Throw in a Crow Pose after your Downward-Facing Dog to get those biceps in shape. Mix it up; combine slow and fast moves, and when the last pose, Savasana (Corpse Pose), arrives, you'll revisit the totally relaxed groove you're used to.

Continue to do the breathing technique (that you learned on page 21) five days a week for 10 minutes a day.

Your kapha yoga workout schedule looks like this:

Workout 1: 30-Minute Kick Start
Workout 2: 60-Minute Core Moves
Workout 3: 90-Minute Fry Fat on the Mat
(Go to www.theyogabodydiet.com to download music playlists for these workouts.)

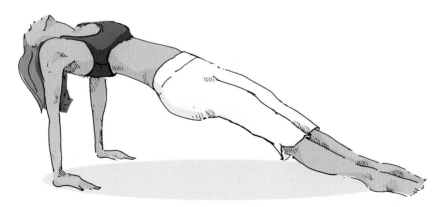

30-Minute Kick Start (Kapha)

POSE NAME	BREATHS (FULL INHALATION AND EXHALATION)	REPS
Cow/Cat	1	4
Cow/Cat Pointer (each side)	1	4
Sun Salutation A	4	3
Plank to Downward-Facing Dog Series	1	5
Sun Salutation A	4	1
Cobra	4	2
Sun Salutation A	4	1
Warrior I (right leg)	4	1
Sun Salutation A	4	1
Warrior I (left leg)	4	1
Sun Salutation A	4	1
Warrior II (right leg)	4	1
Extended Side Angle (right leg)	4	1
Sun Salutation A	4	1
Warrior II (left leg)	4	1
Extended Side Angle (left leg)	4	1
Sun Salutation A	4	1
Eagle (each side)	4	2
Dancer (each side)	4	2
Sun Salutation A	4	1
Double Toe Hold	8	3
Cobbler	5	1
Cow Face (each side)	5	2
Frog	5	1
Bridge	5	3
Windshield Wiper (each side)	5	2
Plow	5	1
Corpse	20	1

TOTAL TIME: 30 MINUTES

60-Minute Core Moves (Kapha)

POSE NAME	BREATHS (FULL INHALATION AND EXHALATION)	REPS
Reclined Cobbler	10	1
Sun Salutation A	4	5
Plank to Downward-Facing Dog	1	10
Sun Salutation B	5	5
Plank to Downward-Facing Dog	1	10
Sun Salutation B	5	1
Warrior II (right leg)	4	1
Sun Salutation B	5	1
Warrior II (left leg)	4	1
Sun Salutation B	5	1
Warrior I (right leg)	4	1
Sun Salutation B	5	1
Warrior I (left leg)	4	1
Sun Salutation B	5	1
Side Plank (each side)	4	2
Sun Salutation B	5	1
Triangle (right side)	4	1
Revolved Triangle (right side)	4	1
Sun Salutation B	5	1
Triangle (left side)	4	1
Revolved Triangle (left side)	4	1
Sun Salutation B	5	1
Tree (right side)	10	1
Tree with Lotus (right side)	10	1
Tree (left side)	10	1
Tree with Lotus (left side)	10	1
Boat	8	1
Reverse Plank	8	1

(continued)

POSE NAME	BREATHS (FULL INHALATION AND EXHALATION)	REPS
Boat	8	1
Reverse Plank	8	1
Pigeon (each side)	10	1
Bridge	8	3
Fish	8	3
Supported Fish	10	1
Corpse	20	1
TOTAL TIME: 60 MINUTES		

90-Minute Fry Fat on the Mat (Kapha)

POSE NAME	BREATHS (FULL INHALATION AND EXHALATION)	REPS
Lotus	10	1
Cow/Cat	4	2
Cow/Cat Pointer (each side)	4	2
Sun Salutation A	9	5
Plank	4	1
Low Pushup	4	1
Plank	4	1
Side Plank (each side)	4	1
Crow	4	2
Sun Salutation B	9	5
Plank	4	1
Low Pushup	4	1
Plank	4	1
Side Plank (each side)	4	1
Crow	4	2
Sun Salutation A	9	5
Warrior II (right leg)	8	1
Reverse Warrior (right leg)	8	1

POSE NAME	BREATHS (FULL INHALATION AND EXHALATION)	REPS
Kneeling Lunge (right leg)	8	1
Warrior III (right leg)	8	1
Downward-Facing Dog	10	1
Pigeon (right leg)	8	1
Sun Salutation A	9	5
Warrior II (left leg)	8	1
Reverse Warrior (left leg)	8	1
Kneeling Lunge (left leg)	8	1
Warrior III (left leg)	8	1
Downward-Facing Dog	8	1
Pigeon (left leg)	8	1
Sun Salutation B	9	5
Bridge with Roll	8	1
Boat	8	1
Bridge with Roll	8	1
Boat	8	1
Camel	8	1
Hero	8	1
Cow Face (each side)	10	1
Pigeon (each side)	10	1
Double Pigeon (each side)	10	1
Frog	10	1
Fish	8	1
Supported Fish	8	1
Shoulder Stand	8	1
Happy Baby	5	1
Reclined Cobbler	5	1
Reclined Twist	5	1
Corpse	20	1
TOTAL TIME: 90 MINUTES		

6

WEEK 4: EAT, SLEEP, AND EXERCISE FOR ALL-DAY ENERGY

What I admire and love is the generous and spontaneous soil which flowers and fruits all seasons.
—Ralph Waldo Emerson

You've spent the past 3 weeks re-educating your body to burn fat. Now, instead of gobbling up every sugar molecule it can find, your body is busy burning its own fat for fuel. Last week, you contributed to this process by eating a large lunch and smaller dinner. When you eat a large lunch and effortlessly make it through the afternoon without hunger, your body is naturally burning fat.

Keep in mind that the key word here is *effortlessly*. The moment you strain to keep from eating, the body's stress response will kick in and demand emergency fuel—in the form of sugar and caffeine—causing you to store the very fat you're trying to burn. Just like yoga, the diet

is based on the principle of *ahimsa,* or "non-harming." If you encountered any struggle last week, take a step back. You can repeat any of the weeks for as long as you need to, even if that means returning to sipping water and refining your ability to eat slowly and mindfully. That's the best feature of *The Yoga Body Diet:* You will benefit from every part of the plan.

But we're willing to bet that you are feeling absolutely fabulous. In that case, here is what's brewing this week:

1. EAT DINNER EARLIER

The longer you go between meals without eating, the more time your body spends burning fat. That's because when you eat, the body ditches its fat-burning mission to deal with the sugar you just swallowed. But you need to eat, obviously. Not eating sends your body into star-

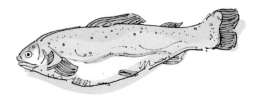

vation mode, which is stressful on all systems and actually results in losing muscle before fat.

However, you can short-circuit these reactions while still providing your body with the nutrients it needs, without feeling starved—or even hungry, for that matter. How? By eating dinner a little earlier. Making this one itsy-bitsy change puts your body in its optimum fat-burning state while you're fast asleep. It couldn't be easier. And get this: You actually sleep better when your body is burning fat instead of digesting carbohydrates. Fat is calm, stable fuel. It is relaxing and sedating. Carbs, on the other hand, hijack your sleep cycles by stirring you awake when blood sugar levels dip. (If you ever wake up starving in the middle of the night, this is why.)

This week, you're going to put meaning back into the word *breakfast*. We encourage you to go at least 12 hours between dinner and breaking the fast the following morning. So, if you normally eat breakfast at 7:00 a.m., make sure you've swallowed the last bite of your last meal for the day by 7:00 p.m. By all means, feel free to go longer than 12 hours if you are able to. However, if this length of time seems daunting, take baby steps. For example, if you currently finish eating for the day by 9:00 p.m. and are chowing on breakfast at 6:00 a.m., extend the amount of time between the two meals by one hour per day. So, keeping breakfast at the same time, finish eating by 8:00 p.m. one day, 7:00 p.m. the next, and 6:00 p.m. the next. Then, either continue finishing by 6:00 p.m. or take it back one more hour to 5:00 p.m. for the remaining days. Remember: This should be effortless and struggle-free. Here are some other tips to make it easier.

Going for the Long Haul

This diet is about forging a beautiful connection between your body and your mind, and it's up to you to honor that relationship. You may be surprised to learn that during Week 4 your body may tell you that it doesn't need dinner. Your body is wise. Listen to it. (By the same token, it may be saying, "Feed me more!" in which case we also encourage you to listen and feed it larger portions.)

You may find that you're willing to forego dinner or that you are simply not hungry at dinnertime because you have been burning food throughout the day, slowly and methodically. Keep in mind that this is not a goal, a principle, or a requirement. (We're looking at you, pittas.) Skip dinner only if you don't want it. This may happen only once or not at all. Check in with your body at the dinnertime you have set for yourself. If you are hungry, eat. If you don't eat when you're hungry, you will stress yourself out and counteract all of the fat burning that's been happening. But if you are not hungry, skip dinner and go to bed earlier. Your body will spend even more time in its fat-burning zone.

De-Stress Your Diet

VATA

Stress: "Twelve hours without eating? I want a nighttime snack!"

Solution: First, look at how long you're going between eating dinner and bedtime. If it's more than 3 hours (for example, if you finish eating dinner at 7:00 p.m. and aren't going to bed until 11:00 p.m.), that may be the reason you feel hungry. Having trouble falling asleep earlier than you're used to? Try taking a warm bath or shower right before bed. When you step out, the cool air dials down your inner thermostat, mimicking the naturally cooler temperature your body reaches when you're sleeping. You may also find that drinking a mug of herbal tea with a few drops of honey is calming and satisfying.

PITTA

Stress: "I woke up at 2:00 a.m. and I was wide awake!"

Solution: Be careful of the tendency to feast yourself to sleep. While eating before bed may seem like a good way to invite deep sleep, food can actually function as a stimulant. Instead of completing the digestion and burning fat all night, your sugar supply runs out hours after you fall asleep; and when internal sirens go off, you wake up alert and on the hunt for more sugar. The deep reserves of fat we use to fuel bodily functions while asleep are not there. Avoid snacks that hamper shut-eye by consuming more at dinner. If your stomach is still speaking to you before bedtime, sip hot water and honey 20 minutes before bed. If worst comes to worst, have a handful of nuts before you retire. Over time, wean yourself from the nuts by making the time you eat them earlier and in smaller quantities. As a result you will sleep cleaner, sounder, and longer.

KAPHA

Stress: "I can't believe this is working."

Solution: This is not exactly a problem, if you ask us. Kaphas are unlikely to encounter many challenges this week, because they naturally metabolize food more slowly than the rest of us and are able to go longer stretches of time without eating. Our advice, however, is this: Recognize when you feel full and stop eating. This will prevent your tendency to overeat simply out of habit or the desire to please those around you.

1. Remember to sip water throughout the day. You will find it especially helpful to drink 8 ounces of water every hour following lunch. This helps to cleanse the body. It will also make you feel full. At this stage, the water can be either warm, or at room temperature, which is easier to drink in large quantities.

2. Adjust your bedtime. The state of Americans' sleep habits is a nightmare. On average, we sleep a mere 6 hours and 40 minutes per night during the week, but most of us need as many as 8 or 9 hours to feel fully rested. Plus, the more you skimp on sleep, the harder it becomes to balance out the sleep debt you accrue. No wonder we're walking around like zombies from *Night of the Living Dead*.

If you feel hungrier when you're sleep-deprived, it isn't all in your head. Well, maybe it *is* in your head, when you consider that sleep deprivation causes levels of ghrelin, a hormone that tells you to eat more, to rise; and leptin, which tells you to stop eating, to fall. Not only do you feel hungrier, but, as a University of Chicago study found, people who slept for only 4 hours per night, two nights in a row, craved foods that were high in sugar, salt, starch, and—no surprise here—calories. Another study found that people who got enough sleep were also more likely to make healthier food choices.

Right off the bat, getting enough sleep each night can protect your body from the stressors that cause poor eating habits. But let's be realistic: having dinner at 6:00 p.m. and staying up for 6 more hours isn't going to work. Of course you'll get hungry. But move bedtime up a couple of hours, to, say, 9:00 p.m., and it will be a seamless change to make. You will literally be losing weight in your sleep.

2. DO THREE YOGA WORKOUTS A WEEK

Week 3 was about stability. In Week 4, we want to keep what works and spend our energy on making it stick. What does that mean for yoga for your type? It means you should stick to the three workouts a week we outlined in Chapter 5. If you've found an at-home routine that has you feeling energized and toned and optimistic, keep it up.

Ultimately, the goal for this week is three yoga sessions. Maybe to get three workouts in, you need to put yourself in the hands of a capable teacher. Part of this week is finding the formula that works for you. We want to make this easy, so we've designed at-home workouts, but studio practices can be energizing. We recommend that when you are ready, you have a teacher check in on you at least once a month.

Finding a Yoga Class

If you're a pitta, you're probably thinking, "There's got to be more to this diet than this." If you're kapha, you'd probably like to see the week's formula stay the same as Week 1. Vatas may be unsure how to stick to the plan outlined thus far. Whatever your dosha, Week 4 is a good time in the program to get out of your comfort zone. If you haven't already, it's time to find a yoga studio, a teacher, and a class or two that work for you.

It's up to us to seek the support we need to improve our yoga practice by finding the right studio, teacher, and schedule. If you can get these three factors to work for you, you'll not only have supervision and feedback from someone with more experience or insightful observations, but you'll ward off common alignment errors, potential yoga injuries, and feelings of malaise or boredom. Here are a few tips that can help you find a good fit.

• **You don't need special gear.** Anyone who tells you that need the $100 yoga mat is crazy. The essential "gear" includes a mat (rentable at every studio for about $2.00 or so) and clothing (you already own something that will suffice). If you attend 20 classes, that's about equal to buying your first mat, so if you see 20 or more classes in your future, consider buying a mat to call your own. As for clothes, something that won't bare your undergarments will work. Any pant without a gaping waistband and typical workout clothing like a sports bra and a tight-fitting tank will do the trick.

• **Treat your first class like a blind date**. You don't have to go back. Yes, we know the agony of finding a class that fits your schedule and commute only to have it let you down, but the trick is to see the search itself as a part of yoga. Be honest about how you'd feel coming back. If you are only lukewarm, it didn't work for you. If your body feels amazing 24 hours later, there is a lot at that class for you.

• **Ask around**. Often, talented teachers have a good reputation. They're worth finding. Because so many studios employ teachers who teach all over, call the front desk and explain what you're looking for, as in, "I'm new to yoga but I want a hard, sweaty class." Ask the desk attendant what he'd recommend. You can even say, "I really want to do more inversions; does anyone spend a lot of time teaching those?" We recommend you get a "spiritual debrief." If chanting or meditating make you uncomfortable, say so upfront: "I don't want anything preachy. I know it's not mandatory, but can you recommend a class that puts the emphasis more on the poses and less on the philosophy?" Interview the yoga school or teacher like you would a babysitter or a future employee. If you have the right chemistry, then when you unroll your mat, you'll feel welcome.

• **Don't get hung up on the style of yoga**. Some studios spit out complicated schedules of classes with sassy names for the styles and levels of yoga. Finding the style for you is an organic process, guided mostly on the teaching style and the convenience of getting to class.

Here are the most common styles of yoga. Keep in mind that different teachers will bring his or her own interpretation to the practice, so avoid getting stuck on one style. Explore.

• Iyengar: An old classic that regulates its teachers well and will ensure you are always in capable hands. Classes are heavy on alignment instructions and good for anyone with injuries.

• Anusara: A lighter approach to postures that focuses on freeing movements and simple, heart-centric positions.

• Bikram/hot yoga: Yoga in a heated environment that makes for a steamy set of poses you repeat twice. It's simple, clear, and athlete-friendly.

• Kundalini: This term refers to the coil of energy in your spine. These classes aim to unleash dormant energy.

• Hatha: Refers to all yoga, because hatha means matching breath to movement.

• Vinyasa: Means flow, so it'll be fast.

• Restorative: A slower pace. Most classes use props in long, supported poses.

• Power Yoga: Athletic in nature, with sequences that make you strong and sweaty while giving your core muscles a run for their money.

• **DVDs work, too**. The most common question we're asked is what DVDs people can do at home. If you need some motivation but want to take the pressure off yourself to parse out the poses, turn on the TV or go online and research the DVDs and podcasts from these seasoned experts:

• Seane Corn

• Baron Baptiste

• Anna Forrest

• Rodney Yee

• Kelly Morris

• Yoga to the People

Many of us approach yoga class as if we have to fit in, but the truth is, if a teacher or a studio doesn't extend themselves to welcome you, it might not be the best class. Luckily, yoga studios and yoga teachers are plentiful in this day and age. Explore until you find one that's right for you.

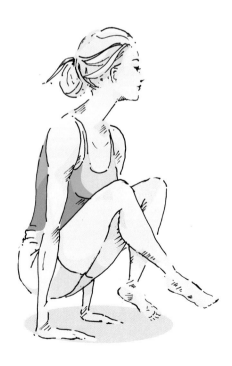

7

MAINTENANCE: YOUR YOGA BODY FOR LIFE

Namaste.
—in Sanskrit, a word used like hello that means "may the light in me greet the light in you"

Gently bow your head in acknowledgement of your success over the past 4 weeks. Externally, you began to eat for whole-body health, picking foods and sticking to routines that promote health and weight loss. You powered up your body's innate fat-burning potential by simply shifting how and what you eat. You gained insight into who you are and how to make balance happen for you. You reinvented your diet using whole foods that encourage calm and balance. And you stood up to your personal stressors using a positive approach: food and fitness.

Perhaps you found your way into your very first Downward-Facing Dog, or you nailed familiar poses that you felt were made for your body and personality type. You learned about the ancient Indian science of Ayurveda and familiarized yourself with ways that the fundamentals fit into your daily life. As a result, you're feeling fresh. The yoga body you've built is part mind, body, *and* spirit.

As we mentioned up front, the effects of *The Yoga Body Diet* are both superficial and profound. If you experienced trouble sleeping before, by now you should be drifting off more easily, sleeping more soundly, and waking up more restored. While the stressors in your life today may be exactly what they were 4 weeks ago, you're finding it easier to remain comfortably in the calm eye of the storm. Your skin is clearer. Your mood is more stable. And digestive issues—heartburn, constipation, and diarrhea—have been resolved. You're looking good externally because you renovated a bit internally.

Coveting a perky yoga butt and trying to find a little more peace in your life are very different goals, but both are perfect in that they got you this far. And because we want to keep growing, it's time to ask, what's next?

If you have more weight to lose, continue eating for your dosha until your have reached a healthy goal weight. Or if you feel unusually moody or sense a life change coming on like a stress tsunami, stay on your dosha-balancing diet. Unlike the commercial programs out there, the dosha diets don't involve deprivation. That means they're safe and healthy to continue long-term.

If you want to go deeper, here's how to maintain a yoga body for life.

The Yoga Body Maintenance Plan

A yoga body isn't made overnight. Think about the people you know who have yoga bodies—Christie Turlington, Reese Witherspoon, your sister-in-law. They've probably worked on and off the mat for years to create their trim physique and healthy glow. Following the Yoga Body Maintenance Plan Principles will keep you on this path while adding more variety to your diet. Here are the four principles to keep in mind when it comes to building a yoga body for life.

1. Continue following the Week 1 guidelines

2. Eat for the seasons.

3. Detox twice a year.

4. Deepen your yoga practice.

Maintenance Principle 1: Continue following the Week 1 guidelines

By now you have seen how important eating properly is to weight loss. (Eating properly for a yoga body means, of course, eating three meals per day, making lunch bigger than dinner, and limiting distractions during mealtime.) You also saw how the Week 1 guidelines provide unique physical and mental benefits for your dosha. They continue to play a major role in keeping the weight off. That's because eating regular, satisfying meals fires up your metabolism while staving off hunger pangs. At the same time, controlling distractions (silencing your phone, stepping away from e-mail, and turning off the TV) prevents mindless eating. When you eat this way the majority of the time, your meals get digested and eliminated properly. Slip-ups take less of a toll on the progress you've made because your body is in peak fat-burning shape.

Maintenance Principle 2: Eat for the seasons

Eating seasonal harvests not only accomplishes the task of keeping your weight stable but supports the environment and economy, saves you money, and effortlessly detoxifies you.

In Ayurveda, each dosha correlates with a season. It's no accident that the constitutions of each type mirror the properties of the seasons:

- Vata constitutions are cold, like winter.

- Pitta constitutions are hot, like summer.

- Kapha constitutions are associated with moisture and with springtime.

The same diets that pacify doshic imbalances can provide balance for everyone—no matter your dosha—during those specific times of the year. It is also no accident that the diets that balance each dosha are based on the foods nature provides during the dosha's corresponding season. So, for instance, the pitta diet favors fresh fruits and vegetables, abundant during the summer's long growing season. Similarly, the vata diet emphasizes high-fat, high-protein foods, which are plentiful during the cold winter. And of course, spring provides a bounty of greens and sprouts, foods integral to the kapha diet.

According to Ayurveda, eating with the seasons naturally creates balance and weight maintenance year-round. What this means is that after the weight-loss project is out of the way, during the winter you'll follow the vata diet, in the summer eat the pitta diet, and in the spring follow the kapha diet.

What about fall? Technically, we consume the nuts, grains, and root vegetables harvested in the fall growing season during the winter, when the earth provides little. The fall months are split between the summer (pitta) diet early on, when the weather is still warm, and the winter (vata) diet toward the end of the season, when the mercury drops. Ayurveda suggests that we actually harvest food in only three seasons of the year; and typically, winter is a season of rest even for nature—so there are harvests in spring, summer, and fall. The late fall harvest supports us through the winter. Dr. Douillard's previous book, *The 3-Season Diet*, explains how to eat seasonally and goes into depth about the resulting health benefits. Specifically, here's how the year breaks down:

• Follow the kapha (spring) diet in March, April, May, and June.

• Follow the pitta (summer) diet in July, August, September, and October.

• Follow the vata (winter) diet in November, December, January, and February.

The wonderful thing about eating for the seasons is that no food is off limits. This means you'll never feel restricted. You can eat every-thing—just wait for the appropriate time of year. And the more closely you follow each diet during its respective season, the more you'll begin to crave the types of foods emphasized during each time of year. The truth is, you probably already hanker for warm soups and stews in the winter; salads in the spring; and fresh, juicy fruits in the summer.

When eating for the seasons, be mindful of two things. First, follow the diet that correlates with your dosha particularly closely during that dosha's season. A vata can easily slip out of balance during the cold, dry winter months. But the vata diet provides warm, moisturizing foods to help vatas maintain balance during that time of the year. The same goes for pittas during the summer and kaphas during the spring. This also means that once a year you will automatically recalibrate, if needed, and drop pounds that may have crept up on you if you weren't paying attention to what you were eating.

The second thing to remember is this: Do not abandon the central principles of your dosha's diet even when eating for the seasons. If you're a pitta, you know that you should minimize spices, but spices are plentiful in the spring diet. While it's fine to use more spices during the spring than you would during the hot summer (and it's also okay to enjoy many of the spicy dishes you love), try to consume spices in moderation. For example, have one spicy meal per week and use just a sprinkle of spices when cooking. Similarly, kapha types know to avoid heavy, oily foods, the very foods that make up the winter (vata) diet. Go ahead and enjoy oils, nuts, and meats during the winter, but keep portions of heavy, oily foods small.

Maintenance Principle 3:
Detox twice a year

In Chapter 1, you saw that stress causes a thick mucus to form along your intestines, clogging your body's ability to properly digest fats and other nutrients from your diet, resulting in tummy troubles, cravings, and ultimately, weight gain. Eating properly, as well as eating for your dosha, will strip away this film.

But there's more. Toxins—heavy metals, carcinogens, preservatives, and pesticides, among others—find their way into your body. They're all around us, in the air we breathe, the water we drink, and the foods we eat. Certain toxins, called free radicals, even occur naturally through processes like digestion and breathing.

Your body is equipped with its own detox system, as your organs work every minute of every day to eliminate the toxic waste from metabolism and from chemicals in the environment. But your organs can get overloaded—and stress slows this process even more. When this happens, toxins circulate through your bloodstream, lodging themselves in fat cells (including those in your brain!). They chip away at your body's defenses, at first causing issues such as allergies, rashes, headaches, colds, depression, PMS, and more—ultimately leading to disease.

The solution? Detox for four days twice a year.

Detoxification was a crucial part of optimal health even 5,000 years ago, when Ayurveda was in its infancy. Back then, environmental toxins were minimal, and yet detoxification played a huge role in an Ayurvedic prescription for optimal health. Today, with an extremely toxic environment, detoxification has again become a requirement for optimal health.

Ayurveda suggests a comprehensive detox called *panchakarma*, in which patients retreat for a week or more to purify and rejuvenate the mind, body, spirit, and emotions. Patients receive 2 to 3 hours of Ayurvedic therapy, with two therapists, individualized yoga, breathing, and meditation for up to 5 hours a day, with a special diet, self-inquiry, emotional release, and even the option of staying in silence. Dr. Douillard has been administering panchakarma since 1987. Studies on panchakarma have shown that 13 of the major cancer-causing fat-soluble chemical toxins were purged from fats cells during the treatment and continued to be expelled for 3 months after the therapy ended. Extremely toxic chemicals such as dioxin were pulled out of people's fat cells, where they sometimes had been stored for 20 years.

This is why it is so important for us to reset our ability to burn fat. It is not only for weight loss; it is an essential component of good health. The detox we describe here is actually used as a preparatory part of the panchakarma and has been time-tested for thousands of years as a simple and effective detox program. As with any detox, please consult your doctor before you begin.

There are plenty of extreme detox programs out there that promise to sweep your innards clean. Their methods are by and large unhealthy. They rob you of crucial nutrients and essentially put your body into starvation mode. That is certainly not what we are after here. The goal of the *Yoga Body* Detox is to encourage your body to rid itself of fat cells in which toxins have taken up residence. (Yes, fat is toxic in more ways than one.) You're going to remind your body what it was built to do: Absorb what it needs, and eliminate what it doesn't. The detox is a loving shove in the right direction.

When Do I Detox?

During the spring and fall, or before the onset of seasonal symptoms. The best times to detox are when the earth is doing the same: in the spring (April) and fall (October). In the spring, the earth is rapidly turning over new growth and new life. And, in the fall, the earth is letting go of the fruits of its labor. (Think of an apple releasing from a tree.) If you typically suffer from specific symptoms during certain times of the year (say, springtime allergies, or depression in the winter), detox approximately one month before those symptoms take root, and see what happens. The toxins themselves are partly to blame for your symptoms. And a buildup of toxins can interfere with your body's ability to properly absorb nutrients from foods. A deficiency of certain nutrients—even if they're in your diet but aren't getting assimilated into your body—may be the culprit behind seasonal woes. Cleansing will remedy this.

This cleanse is not going to leave you feeling depleted. You are not going to be starving or chugging some crazy juice concoction. You are still going to be eating three daily meals. Having said that, it's important to take some time for yourself while cleansing. What good are your efforts if you're still whizzing through your day at a million miles per hour, completely stressed out? Your digestive system is going to miss the message that it's time to chill out and let go. As you reset your digestive system through the detox, it pays to reset your mind, too. If possible, detox when you are able to take a few days off from work or at least when things at work have settled down, such as between deadlines. For 4 days, give yourself permission to relax.

Directions for the 4-Day Detox

IMPORTANT NOTE: Do not do this if you have gallbladder issues or trouble digesting fat. If you have any doubts about whether to proceed, please consult your medical practitioner.

1. First thing in the morning, drink ghee (clarified butter) or flaxseed oil. See Chapter 8 for instructions to make ghee at home.

> ❖ Day 1: 2 teaspoons ghee or flaxseed oil
>
> ❖ Day 2: 4 teaspoons ghee or flaxseed oil
>
> ❖ Day 3: 6 teaspoons ghee or flaxseed oil
>
> ❖ Day 4: 8 teaspoons ghee or flaxseed oil

Why ghee? The purpose of this cleanse is to get your body to remove fat cells containing toxins. During these 4 days, you're going to be eating a nonfat diet *except for ghee*. Consuming it first thing in the morning automatically puts your body in fat-burning mode and keeps it there. Because you won't be ingesting any other fat, your body turns to its own fat cells for fuel.

If you have trouble stomaching ghee, mix it with soymilk and drink quickly. As an alternative, mix 1 tablespoon of flaxseed oil with $\frac{1}{2}$ cup of cottage cheese. This combination has an effect similar to that of ghee, but it contains slightly less fat, so it won't give your body as big a metabolic jumpstart. Wait at least 30 minutes after you have your morning ghee or flaxseed oil before eating breakfast.

2. Eat a nonfat diet. Now that your metabolism is revved up, you're going to feed it a zero-fat diet. Continue eating your three daily meals. Keep drinking your warm water, which is especially crucial here. Doing so helps flush those fat cells and toxins out of your system.

What should I eat?

Breakfast: Nonfat cooked cereal, such as steel-cut oatmeal or cream of wheat. Egg whites with vegetables. Fresh seasonal fruit if you want it.

Lunch and dinner: Brown rice with black beans (see page 116 for recipe) is going to be your go-to meal this week. Remember, it's only 4 days, so even if you eat them every day, sometimes twice a day, it will get only so boring. Brown rice with black beans is based on an Indian diet staple called *kicharee*, which is essentially pureed rice and beans with powerful spices. The taste and texture (not far from baby food) are challenging for Westerners, but a dish of plain rice and beans works equally well. The combination is ideal for keeping blood sugar stable because they're high in fiber, so they are digested slowly; and beans provide the protein you need for energy. Other possible go-to meals are nonfat vegetable soup (such as minestrone) and salad with nonfat dressing (such as a squeeze of lemon and drop of honey).

3. Drink 1 ½ cups prune juice on the evening of the fourth night. Nature's laxative will give your digestive system one more sweep before you welcome a wider variety of foods back into your diet. It goes without saying: You'll want to clear your schedule this evening.

4. Avoid these foods, which interfere with the detox:

- Bread, crackers, or any baked goods

- Meats, fats, and oily foods (such as butter, yogurt, nuts, oils, cheese, pizza)

- Sprouts, pickles, and vinegar

- Cold drinks, cold foods, caffeine, and alcohol

- White sugar

- Creamy or spicy foods

Maintenance Principle 4: Deepen your yoga practice

Like anything else you've dedicated yourself to in the past—where dieting and exercising are concerned—you know that when you stop doing them, you stop benefiting from them. And you know there are plateaus in health and in life.

Yoga is no different. The more you build your yoga body, the more you strengthen your mind, sculpt your biceps, tighten your butt, and flatten your belly. If you already have a regular yoga practice, keep at it. We recommend a minimum of 3 hours total per week, to begin. When stress is under control, you'll see that with the absence of tension, the mind and body begin to crave more of this relaxed state.

What exactly does the phrase "deepen your practice" mean? It simply means "explore." Meditation may be your next adventure. A weekend workshop at a local retreat center may work, or you may buy a DVD and learn more at home. We haven't talked much about meditation, but on the following pages we'll give you a brief introduction as a way to dip your toe into the practice and see how it feels.

Why Meditation?

Yoga poses, especially the sweaty sequences versions now beloved in the West, actually grew out of meditation practice in the ancient East. Yoga was invented as a reaction to a culture's inability to meditate. The people who sat and stilled their minds were getting distracted. Commerce had arrived, and their monk-like discipline was waning, while the marketplace began to thrive. As a reaction to the loss of discipline, systems of exercise were created that burned off mental and physical tension in order to allow the meditator to sit better and longer.

Set Your Intention

No, you don't have to meditate to be a true yogi. Yes, you should try. If you've come this far, you may actually be in a place where you are ready for something new.

So, let's approach the practice with complete and utter openness. Here is a simple but perfect sequence that warms up your body prior to meditation.

We've experienced profound change simply by taking time to look at how we breathe and eat. If we continue to become skilled in our ability to sit still and encourage balance in our minds and bodies, we'll be better for it. According to yoga, anything's possible if you truly mind the body.

Namaste.

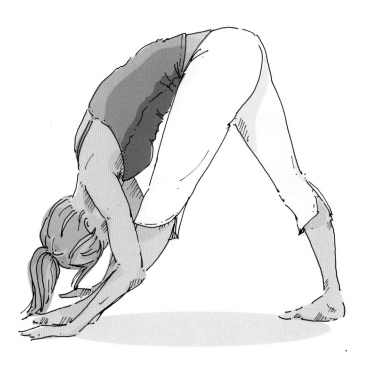

Pre-Meditation Sequence

Sometimes it's nice to warm up your body before moving into meditation. The warm-up should last 5 minutes or until your spine feels warmer and more limber than when you started. Choose one of the three options below depending on your goals. No matter which sequence you choose, you will end in Corpse in preparation for meditation.

1. BURN FAT (Hold each pose for 10 breaths.)

Plank
Rock 'n' Roll Pushup (both sides)
Dolphin
Crow

2. GAIN ENERGY (Hold each pose for 20 breaths on each side.)

Triangle
Pigeon
Cow Face

3. RESTORE (Hold each pose for a full 5 minutes.)

Reclined Cobbler
Reclined Fish
Legs Up the Wall

Meditation

When you are finished with your pre-meditation sequence, move into Corpse Pose until your back is relaxed and you feel your spine and the muscles parallel to the spine really go soft. Keep your throat open, your jaw relaxed, and the space between your eyebrows soft. Stay here for 10 breaths to 5 minutes.

Come to Sit

Rolling onto your right side, use your hands to push up to a seated position, ankles crossed.

Meditate

Your body has been relaxed by the above poses. Now, let's take it a step further.

Sit comfortably in a cross-legged position.

(continued)

Start with one round of Alternate Nostril Breathing (see opposite page), as it's believed to balance out the activity in the two lobes of the brain. It is calming and stabilizes your mood.

Use a timer; when you are comfortable, set it for 18 minutes, and begin.

1. In the cross-legged sitting position, place your hands in your lap, palms up, one on top of the other. The top palm should be the opposite palm from the ankle crossed in front.

2. Soften the space between your eyebrows.

3. Let your jaw go slack.

4. Close your eyelids gently.

5. Tune in to the feeling of your breath above your upper lip.

6. Release any remaining tension in your face and the rest of your body.

7. Repeat to yourself silently, eight to ten times, the mantra *om namah shivaya* (pronounced ohm–nah–ma–sha–vay–ah) as if it were a gentle lullaby.

What are you saying? "I bow to the divine in myself." It's simply a way to acknowledge that you want to look inside yourself. Don't make it heavy. If another word or phrase works better for you, use that instead.

- Let the words or sounds lull you into a calmer, quieter mental state. If thoughts come into your head, acknowledge them but let them go. Don't get distracted by the grocery list or feel badly that you thought of it; just send it in another direction.

- Withdraw from the sensory experience you just had by focusing on the soft words in your head until they become white noise. Then, when you know you are ready to let go further and think nothing, let the mantra drift away, and simply sit quietly.

- See what comes.

- When the timer dings, slowly open your eyes. If you need more time, stay.

- To ground your energy, fold forward over your legs, taking a few deep breaths.

- Roll up, exercising your spine while tuning in to the physical sensations around you.

- Enjoy the new sense of calm and peace throughout your mind and body.

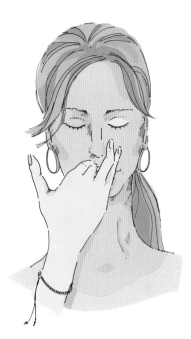

Alternate Nostril Breathing

1. Place the palm of your right hand to face up.

2. Draw your pointer and middle finders into your palm, leaving the ring finger, pinky, and thumb extended.

3. Drag your ring finger down the outer edge of the left side of the bridge of your nose, ending above the nostril opening at the end of the cartilage.

4. Use the ring finger of your right hand to close your left nostril.

5. Close your eyes and inhale through the right nostril for four counts.

6. Use your thumb to close the right nostril.

7. Simultaneously remove your ring finger from the left nostril and exhale all of your breath out of the left nostril. (This is one-half of the breath.)

8. Keeping your thumb on your right nostril, inhale through your left nostril for four counts.

9. Close your left nostril using your ring finger.

10. Simultaneously remove your thumb from your right nostril and exhale all of your breath using the right nostril. (This is the second half of the breath.)

11. Repeat the full breath three times to complete one full round.

12. Work toward completing six rounds, or 18 breaths (three full breaths, six times).

8

RECIPES

I was 32 when I started cooking; up until then, I just ate.
—Julia Child

Choosing foods that balance your dosha may seem like an overwhelming task. The solution is right here. Vatas, how do whole wheat crêpes with lemon-ricotta filling sound? What do you pittas think of pineapple coconut fried rice? Kaphas, are you in the mood for a chicken-mushroom quesadilla with chipotle-lime corn salsa? If your mouth is watering, join the club.

Each recipe has three versions: one for vata, one for pitta, and one for kapha. Each is carefully crafted to use the very best foods for each type while providing a slew of nutritional benefits. What's more, most of these recipes can be made in 30 minutes or less, so you can quickly whip them up during a hectic weekday night. Despite their fancy-sounding names, they don't require any fancy cooking methods, tools, or hard-to-find ingredients. Most require only a handful of fresh ingredients (no preservatives!) located along the perimeter of your favorite grocery store, as well as herbs and spices that you already have in your kitchen. Each meal contains the right balance of fat, protein, and carbohydrates, so they'll be digested slowly; and, as a result, keep your blood sugar levels stable and your hunger in check.

In short, we blended principles from the science of Ayurveda with the knowledge of Western nutritional science to provide the maximum benefit in every bite. All you have to do is eat!

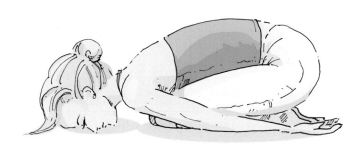

The Yoga Body Diet and Organics

Buy organic ingredients whenever possible. Organic produce is grown without the pesticides, herbicides, and fungicides used in conventional farming. Animals raised organically are given foods free of antibiotics, added hormones, and other drugs. (You are what *they* eat, too!) Eating organic fruits, vegetables, grains, dairy, and meats means avoiding questionable additives that could harm your body.

Not only is organic food healthier for you, it is also healthier for the earth. Chemicals used in conventional farming pollute the environment and can also contaminate local bodies of water, harming marine wildlife and possibly affecting our fresh-water supply. Organic farms, on the other hand, keep local ecosystems intact and do not use pesticides or other chemicals that can leach into the groundwater or make their way into our lakes, rivers, and oceans.

Two other guidelines to keep in mind when shopping for ingredients are to buy local, and buy in season. Locally grown foods have minimal impact on the environment as they do not have to be transported very far to make their way into your refrigerator. Furthermore, food that is in season is the most nutritious. (Nutrition content of fruits and vegetables declines the longer they sit around waiting to be consumed.) The single best way to fill your diet with locally grown seasonal foods? Frequent the farmers' market—that's the only kind of food you'll find there.

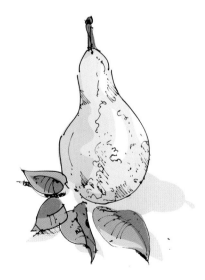

BREAKFAST

Homemade Granola

Granola is a delicious way to get whole grains into your diet. Whole grains have been shown to reduce your risk of heart disease, possibly help prevent cancer, and help control your weight. Although tasty, many store-bought granolas are packed with fat, preservatives, and sugar—things you won't miss once you taste this homemade version! Each of these versions contains the best nuts, dried fruits, seeds, sweeteners, and spices for your type.

Makes five ½-cup servings

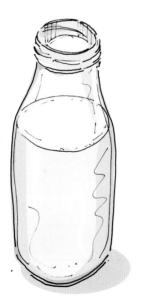

Vata

- 2 cups rolled oats
- ¼ cup water
- 2 tablespoons maple syrup
- 2 tablespoons ground flaxseeds
- 1 tablespoon canola oil
- 1 teaspoon cinnamon
- ½ teaspoon ground cardamom
- ¼ cup chopped hazelnuts
- ¼ cup chopped dates
- 1 cup soy milk

Preheat the oven to 375°F. Coat a large baking sheet (with sides) with cooking spray. Set aside. Place the oats, water, maple syrup, flaxseeds, oil, cinnamon, and cardamom in a large bowl. Stir well to combine. Spread evenly on the baking sheet and bake for 20 minutes, stirring carefully once or twice. Add the hazelnuts and dates, and bake an additional 5 minutes. Remove and cool completely before storing in an airtight container at room temperature for up to 1 week. Serve with soy milk.

Pitta

- 2 cups rolled oats
- ¼ cup water
- 2 tablespoons maple syrup
- 2 tablespoons ground flaxseeds
- 1 tablespoon vanilla extract
- 1 tablespoon sunflower oil
- 1 teaspoon cinnamon
- ½ teaspoon ground cardamom
- ¼ cup unsweetened flaked coconut
- ¼ cup pumpkin seeds
- 1 cup soy milk

Preheat oven to 375°F. Coat a large baking sheet (with sides) with cooking spray. Set aside. Place the oats, water, maple syrup, flaxseeds, vanilla extract, oil, cinnamon, and cardamom in a large bowl. Stir well to combine. Spread evenly on the baking sheet and bake for 20 minutes, stirring carefully once or twice. Add the coconut and pumpkin seeds, and bake an additional 5 minutes. Remove and cool completely before storing in an airtight container at room temperature for up to 1 week. Serve with soy milk.

Kapha

(best served with heated milk)

- 2 cups rolled oats
- ¼ cup water
- 1 tablespoon molasses
- 2 tablespoons ground flaxseeds
- 1 tablespoon corn oil
- 1 teaspoon cinnamon
- ½ teaspoon ground cardamom
- ¼ teaspoon ground cloves
- 2 tablespoons dried cranberries
- 2 tablespoons raisins
- 1 cup soy milk

Preheat oven to 375°F. Coat a large baking sheet (with sides) with cooking spray. Set aside. Place the oats, water, molasses, flaxseeds, oil, cinnamon, cardamom, and cloves in a large bowl. Stir well to combine. Spread evenly onto the baking sheet and bake for 20 minutes, stirring carefully once or twice. Add the dried cranberries and raisins, and bake an additional 5 minutes. Remove and cool completely before storing in an airtight container at room temperature for up to 1 week. Serve with warm soy milk

Light-As-Air Crêpes

These airy crêpes are made with heart-healthy, unprocessed whole grain flour. The fillings contain antioxidant-rich berries, which strengthen the pancreas and stabilize blood sugar levels.

Makes 14 crêpes (2 per serving)

Vata

Crêpes

  1 cup whole wheat flour

1½ cups soy milk

  3 egg whites

  2 tablespoons canola oil

 ¼ teaspoon salt

Filling

  1 cup fresh berries, such as raspberries or blueberries

 ¼ cup water

  2 tablespoons raw honey

  1 cup reduced-fat ricotta cheese

  1 teaspoon grated lemon zest

Place the flour, soy milk, egg whites, oil, and salt in a blender or food processor, and blend until a smooth batter forms. There should be no lumps. Cover and refrigerate for at least 1 hour or up to 8 hours.

Coat a pancake griddle or crêpe pan with cooking spray. Heat over medium-high heat. Pour 3 tablespoons of the batter into the griddle or pan. If using a crêpe pan, immediately tilt and gently rotate the pan to coat the entire bottom. If using a griddle, spread out the batter with the back of a large spoon or measuring cup. Cook until the edges begin to turn brown and small bubbles form on the surface of the crêpe. Loosen the edges and flip the crêpe. Cook 15 to 20 seconds more, and transfer to a plate. Repeat for the remaining batter. Stack the crêpes on top of each other. Cover with foil to keep warm.

Place the berries in a small saucepan with the water. Cook over high heat until the berries start to break apart. Remove from the heat and cool 5 minutes before stirring in 1 tablespoon of the honey. Set aside. Combine the ricotta, the remaining honey, and the lemon zest in a food processor or mini-chopper. Pulse until smooth. Place 1 crêpe on a flat surface. Spread 1 heaping tablespoon of the ricotta filling in the center of the crêpe. Roll into a cigar shape. Top with 2 tablespoons of the cooked berries. Repeat for all the crêpes.

Pitta

Crêpes

  1 cup whole wheat flour

1½ cups soy milk

  2 egg whites

  2 tablespoons canola oil

 ¼ teaspoon salt

Filling

  1 cup fresh berries, such as raspberries or blueberries

 ¼ cup water

  2 tablespoons agave nectar

  1 cup reduced-fat ricotta cheese

  1 teaspoon grated orange zest

Place the flour, milk or soy milk, egg whites, oil, and salt in a blender or food processor, and blend until a smooth batter forms. There should be no lumps. Cover and refrigerate for at least 1 hour or up to 8 hours.

Coat a pancake griddle or crêpe pan with nonstick cooking spray. Heat over medium-high heat. Pour 3 tablespoons of the batter into the griddle or pan. If using a crêpe pan, immediately tilt and gently rotate the pan to coat the entire bottom. If using a griddle, spread out the batter with the back of a large spoon or measuring cup. Cook until the edges begin to turn brown and small bubbles form on the surface of the crêpe. Loosen the edges and flip the crêpe. Cook 15 to 20 seconds more, and transfer to a plate. Repeat for the remaining batter. Stack the crêpes on top of each other. Cover with foil to keep warm.

Place the berries in a small saucepan with the water. Cook over high heat until the berries start to break apart. Remove from heat and cool 5 minutes before stirring in 1 tablespoon of the agave. Set aside. Combine the ricotta, the remaining agave, and the orange zest in a food processor. Pulse until smooth. Place 1 crêpe on a flat surface. Spread 1 heaping tablespoon of the ricotta filling in the center of the crêpe. Roll into a cigar shape. Top with 2 tablespoons of the reserved cooked berries. Repeat for all the crêpes.

Kapha

Crêpes

- ¾ cup spelt flour
- ¼ cup buckwheat flour
- 1½ cups soy milk
- 3 egg whites
- 2 tablespoons sunflower oil
- ½ teaspoon cinnamon
- ¼ teaspoon nutmeg
- ¼ teaspoon salt
- ¼ teaspoon ground cloves

Filling

- 4 cups mixed berries, such as blueberries, strawberries, and raspberries
- ½ cup water
- ¼ cup raw honey

Place the spelt flour, buckwheat flour, soy milk, egg whites, oil, cinnamon, nutmeg, salt, and cloves in a blender or food processor, and blend until a smooth batter forms. There should be no lumps. Cover and refrigerate for at least 1 hour or up to 8 hours.

Coat a pancake griddle or crêpe pan with cooking spray. Heat over medium-high heat. Pour 3 tablespoons of the batter into the griddle or pan. If using a crêpe pan, immediately tilt and gently rotate the pan to coat the entire bottom. If using a griddle, spread out the batter with the back of a large spoon or measuring cup. Cook until the edges begin to turn brown and small bubbles form on the surface of the crêpe. Loosen the edges and flip the crêpe. Cook 15 to 20 seconds more, and transfer to a plate. Repeat for the remaining batter. Stack the crêpes on top of each other. Cover with foil to keep warm.

In a skillet over medium heat, cook the berries for 3 minutes, crushing them with a wooden spoon or heat-resistant spatula. Add the water, and cook until bubbly and thick and the berries break down. Remove from the heat, and cool 5 minutes before stirring in the honey.

Place 1 crêpe on a flat surface. Spread 1 heaping tablespoon of the berry filling in the center of the crêpe and roll into a cigar shape. Top with 2 tablespoons of the reserved berries. Repeat for all the crêpes.

Vegetable Omelet

Most people find it hard to include sufficient produce in their diet. Starting off your day with a serving or two brings you that much closer to meeting your quota. Combining the produce with eggs, which are packed with protein, keeps you feeling fuller longer. In fact, a recent study found that people who eat an egg-based breakfast consume fewer calories throughout the day.

Makes 4 servings

Vata

- 4 egg whites
- 2 whole eggs
- ¼ teaspoon salt
- ¼ teaspoon freshly ground black pepper
- 1 teaspoon chopped cilantro
- 1 teaspoon Ghee (opposite)
- 4 spears asparagus, chopped
- 2 tablespoons diced onion
- ¼ cup diced bell pepper
- ¼ cup diced zucchini

Beat the egg whites, whole eggs, salt, black pepper, and cilantro in a small bowl. Heat the ghee over medium heat in a medium skillet. Add the asparagus, onion, bell pepper, and zucchini, and cook until the vegetables just begin to soften. Add the egg mixture, cover, and cook over medium heat until the eggs have set, approximately 5 minutes. Loosen the edges of the omelet using a heat-resistant spatula, fold in half, and transfer to a plate. Cut into 4 slices and serve immediately.

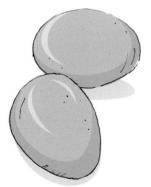

Pitta

- 4 egg whites
- 2 whole eggs
- ¼ teaspoon salt
- ¼ teaspoon freshly ground black pepper
- 1 teaspoon chopped cilantro
- 1 teaspoon Ghee (below)
- 4 spears asparagus, chopped
- 2 tablespoons diced onion
- ¼ cup sliced mushrooms
- ¼ cup diced zucchini

Beat the egg whites, whole eggs, salt, black pepper, and cilantro in a small bowl. Heat the ghee over medium heat in a medium skillet. Add the asparagus, onion, bell pepper, and zucchini, and cook until the vegetables just begin to soften. Add the egg mixture, cover, and cook over medium heat until the eggs have set, approximately 5 minutes. Loosen the edges of the omelet using a heat-resistant spatula, fold in half, and transfer to a plate. Cut into 4 slices and serve immediately.

Kapha

- 4 egg whites
- 2 whole eggs
- ¼ teaspoon salt
- ¼ teaspoon freshly ground black pepper
- 1 teaspoon chopped cilantro
- 1 teaspoon Ghee (below)
- 4 spears asparagus, chopped
- 2 tablespoons diced onion
- ¼ cup sliced mushrooms
- ¼ cup diced bell pepper

Beat the egg whites, whole eggs, salt, black pepper, and cilantro in a small bowl. Heat the ghee over medium heat in a medium skillet. Add the asparagus, onion, bell pepper, and zucchini, and cook until the vegetables just begin to soften. Add the egg mixture, cover, and cook over medium heat until the eggs have set, approximately 5 minutes. Loosen the edges of the omelet using a heat-resistant spatula, fold in half, and transfer to a plate. Cut into 4 slices and serve immediately.

Ghee

Also known as *clarified butter*, ghee is butter that has the milk solids removed during boiling. As a result, it is lower in fat and calories than the real thing, but it can be used for the same purposes, such as spreading on bread or sautéing vegetables. Ghee is acceptable for vata and pitta, but kaphas should use it sparingly, as the kapha diet minimizes fat and dairy.

2 sticks unsalted butter

Place the butter in a medium saucepan over medium-high heat. Bring to a boil, then reduce the heat to medium. The butter will form a foam that will disappear. After 7 to 8 minutes, a second foam will form on top of the butter, and the butter will turn golden. Brown milk solids will be in the bottom of the pan. Gently pour the clarified butter into a heatproof container through a fine mesh strainer or cheesecloth. Store in an airtight container, free from moisture, at room temperature, for up to 1 month.

Makes ¾ cup

Fruit Carpaccio

Each of these fancy (but easy-to-make) salads features the absolute best fruits for your type. Mangoes in the vata recipe are calming to the nervous system, while pineapples are cooling and have anti-inflammatory effects for pitta, and grapefruits have a unique ability to break up mucus, a common kapha complaint.

Makes four 1-cup servings

Vata

1 (½") piece ginger, peeled and chopped
1 tablespoon raw honey
1 teaspoon cinnamon
¼ cup water
2 mangoes
2 peaches

Place the ginger, honey, cinnamon, and water in a blender or mini-chopper. Blend on high until the ginger is well minced. Peel and thinly slice the mangoes, and thinly slice the peaches. Transfer the fruit to a bowl, and pour the drizzle over. Toss to coat, and serve immediately.

Fresh Juices

These fresh juices combine fruits and veggies to provide a wealth of vitamins and minerals that help with everything from making skin glow to building immunity. Not only do they contain superfoods for your dosha, they also have a kick of spice for flavor (ginger for vata and kapha, mint for pitta)—and for additional dosha-balancing benefits.

Makes two 1-cup servings

Vata

2 medium carrots, cut into thirds
1 (½") piece ginger, peeled and cut into thirds
½ cup fresh cherries
½ cup red or green grapes

Place the carrots, ginger, cherries, and grapes in a juicer, and process according to the manufacturer's instructions. Serve immediately.

Pitta

¼ cup water

2 tablespoons packed mint leaves

2 tablespoons packed cilantro leaves

1 tablespoon raw sugar

1 (3"-thick) slice pineapple, thinly sliced (about 2 cups)

¼ large cantaloupe, thinly sliced (about 2 cups)

Place the water, mint, cilantro, and sugar in a blender or mini-chopper, and blend until smooth. Place the pineapple and cantaloupe along with the drizzle in a large bowl. Toss to coat, and serve immediately.

Kapha

2 large grapefruits

2 pints strawberries, stemmed, thinly sliced

¼ cup water

1 tablespoon raw honey

¼ teaspoon ground cloves

¼ teaspoon freshly ground black pepper

With a sharp knife, cut away the rind of the grapefruits. Over a large bowl, cut away the grapefruit segments from the membranes, and allow the juice to drip down into the bowl. Add grapefruit segments and strawberries to the bowl. Add the water, honey, cloves, and pepper and toss, being careful not to break up the grapefruit segments. Serve immediately.

Pitta

1 cup watermelon chunks

½ medium cucumber, peeled and chopped

2 tablespoons packed mint leaves

Place the watermelon, cucumber, and mint in a juicer, and process according to the manufacturer's instructions. Serve immediately.

Kapha

½ head lettuce, cut into 3 pieces

1 apple, cut into quarters

2 medium carrots, cut into thirds

1 (½") piece ginger, peeled and cut into thirds

Place the lettuce, apple, carrots, and ginger in a juicer, and process according to the manufacturer's instructions. Serve immediately.

Chai Tea

Chai, or spiced milk tea, is a drink traditionally savored by yogis and sherpas, but it is now popular in coffee shops everywhere. If you like the store-bought version, this one has the same rich taste, but will be a lot lighter on your waistline—and your wallet.

Makes 2 servings

Vata

1 (1") piece ginger, peeled
2 cups plain soy milk
1 tablespoon freshly brewed fine black tea, such as English Breakfast
1 tablespoon maple syrup

Place all ingredients in small saucepan. Bring to a slow boil. Strain and serve immediately.

Citrus Waffles

The secret ingredient in this recipe is the citrus zest (grapefruit for vata, lemon for pitta, and orange for kapha) because it adds a burst of flavor with virtually zero fat or calories.

Makes 4 servings

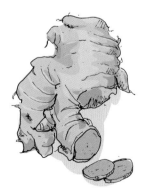

Vata

¾ cup oat flour
¾ cup white whole wheat flour
1 teaspoon baking powder
½ teaspoon baking soda
1 tablespoon raw sugar
¼ teaspoon salt
¾ cup fat-free plain Greek yogurt
Zest of ½ large pink grapefruit
2 tablespoons ghee (page 101)
4 egg whites

Preheat a waffle maker according to the manufacturer's instructions. Place the oat flour, white whole wheat flour, baking powder, baking soda, sugar, and salt in a large bowl. Stir to combine. Add the yogurt, grapefruit zest, and ghee. Stir until just combined.

In another large bowl, beat the egg whites on high speed with an electric mixer until they are fluffy and stiff peaks form. They should cling to the sides of the bowl when you tilt it. Gently fold in the egg whites, one-third at a time. Transfer ½ cup of the batter to the waffle iron. Close the iron, and cook the waffle according to the manufacturer's instructions. Serve immediately. Repeat for all waffles.

Pitta

- 1 (1") piece ginger, peeled
- 2 cups plain soy milk
- 1 tablespoon freshly brewed fine black tea, such as English Breakfast
- 1 tablespoon maple syrup

Place all ingredients in small saucepan. Bring to a slow boil. Strain and serve immediately.

Kapha

- 1 (1") piece ginger, peeled
- 2 cups plain soy milk
- 1 tablespoon freshly brewed fine black tea, such as English Breakfast
- 1 tablespoon raw sugar

Place all ingredients in small saucepan. Bring to a slow boil. Strain and serve immediately.

Pitta

- 1½ cups white whole wheat flour
- 1 teaspoon baking powder
- ½ teaspoon baking soda
- 1 tablespoon raw sugar
- ¼ teaspoon salt
- ¾ cup plain soy milk
  Zest of 1 large lemon
- 2 tablespoons ghee (page 101)
- 4 egg whites

Preheat a waffle maker according to the manufacturer's instructions. Place the flour, baking powder, baking soda, sugar, and salt in a large bowl. Stir to combine. Add the soy milk, lemon zest, and ghee. Stir until just combined.

In another large bowl, beat egg whites on high speed with an electric mixer until they are fluffy and stiff peaks form. They should cling to the sides of the bowl when you tilt it. Gently fold in the egg whites, one-third at a time. Transfer ½ cup of the batter to the waffle iron. Close the iron, and cook the waffle according to the manufacturer's instructions. Serve immediately. Repeat for all waffles.

Kapha

- 1½ cups amaranth flour
- 1 teaspoon baking powder
- ½ teaspoon baking soda
- ¼ teaspoon salt
- 1 tablespoon raw sugar
- ¾ cup fat-free plain Greek yogurt
  Zest of 2 small oranges (about 2 tablespoons)
- 2 tablespoons raisins
- 2 tablespoons ghee (page 101)
- 4 egg whites

Preheat a waffle maker according to the manufacturer's instructions. Place the flour, baking powder, baking soda, sugar, and salt in a large bowl. Stir to combine. Add the yogurt, orange zest, raisins, and ghee. Stir until just combined.

In another large bowl, beat the egg whites on high speed with an electric mixer until they are fluffy and stiff peaks form. They should cling to the sides of the bowl when you tilt it.Gently fold in the egg whites, one-third at a time. Transfer ½ cup of the batter to the waffle iron. Close the iron, and cook the waffle according to the manufacturer's instructions. Serve immediately. Repeat for all waffles.

BERRY PANCAKES

Adding fresh fruit (blueberries for vata, strawberries for pitta, and raspberries for kapha) to pancakes makes them tastier and richer in belly-filling fiber.

Makes 8 pancakes (2 pancakes per serving)

Vata

Blueberry Pancakes

- 1 cup white whole wheat flour
- 2 tablespoons ground flaxseeds
- ½ teaspoon baking powder
- ¼ teaspoon baking soda
- ½ teaspoon ground cinnamon
- ½ teaspoon ground ginger
- ¼ teaspoon freshly ground nutmeg
- ⅛ teaspoon salt
- 1 cup buttermilk
- 1 egg white
- ½ pint blueberries

Preheat the griddle over high heat. Combine the flour, flaxseeds, baking powder, baking soda, cinnamon, ginger, nutmeg, and salt in a large bowl. Make a well in the center, and add the buttermilk and the egg white. Whisk until combined.

Coat the griddle with cooking spray. Pour ¼ cup batter per pancake onto the griddle, and top each one with 6 to 7 blueberries. Cook 3 to 4 minutes, until small bubbles appear on the top. Flip, and cook an additional 3 to 4 minutes, until the pancakes are cooked through. Serve immediately.

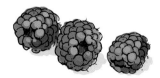

Strawberry Pancakes

- 1 cup white whole wheat flour
- 2 tablespoons ground flaxseeds
- 1/2 teaspoon baking powder
- 1 teaspoon grated orange zest
- 1/4 teaspoon baking soda
- 1/8 teaspoon salt
- 1 cup plain soy milk
- 1 egg white
- 8 strawberries, sliced

Preheat the griddle over high heat. Combine the flour, flaxseeds, baking powder, orange zest, baking soda, and salt in a large bowl. Make a well in the center, and add the soy milk and egg white. Whisk until combined.

Coat the griddle with cooking spray. Pour 1/4 cup batter per pancake onto the griddle, and top each one with the slices from 1 strawberry. Cook 3 to 4 minutes, until small bubbles appear on the top. Flip, and cook an additional 3 to 4 minutes, until the pancakes are cooked through. Serve immediately.

Raspberry Pancakes

- 1/2 cup oat flour
- 1/2 cup buckwheat flour
- 1/2 teaspoon baking powder
- 1/4 teaspoon baking soda
- 1/2 teaspoon ground cinnamon
- 1/4 teaspoon ground cloves
- 1/8 teaspoon salt
- 1 cup buttermilk
- 1 egg white
- 1 tablespoon butter, melted
- 1 tablespoon honey
- 1 cup raspberries

Preheat the griddle over high heat. Combine the oat flour, buckwheat flour, baking powder, baking soda, cinnamon, cloves, and salt in a large bowl. Make a well in the center, and add the buttermilk, egg white, butter, and honey. Whisk until combined.

Coat the griddle with cooking spray. Pour 1/4 cup batter per pancake onto the griddle, and top each one with 3 to 4 raspberries. Cook 3 to 4 minutes, until small bubbles appear on the top. Flip, and cook an additional 3 to 4 minutes, until the pancakes are cooked through. Serve immediately.

FRUIT MUFFINS

Muffins? Yes, please! These are lighter and much healthier for you than the packaged varieties or the kind you get at the coffee shop. Plus, each recipe contains dosha superfoods: warm figs for vata, cooling cherries for pitta, and dried cranberries that counter kapha's tendency to become congested.

Makes 12 muffins (1 muffin per serving)

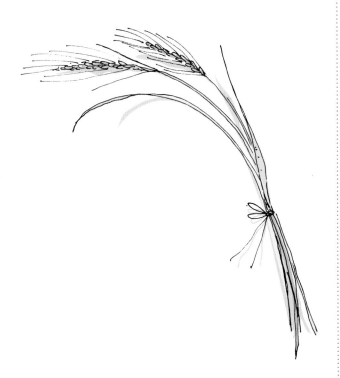

Vata

Lemon-Fig Muffins

 2 cups white whole wheat flour
 1 teaspoon baking powder
 1 teaspoon baking soda
 ½ teaspoon salt
    Zest and juice of 2 lemons
 ⅔ cup raw sugar
 ⅔ cup fat-free milk
 ½ cup canola oil
 2 egg whites
 1 tablespoon vanilla extract
 1 cup chopped dried figs, soaked in hot
    water and drained

Preheat the oven to 325°F. Line a 12-cup muffin pan with paper liners.

Whisk together the flour, baking powder, baking soda, and salt in a medium bowl. Add the lemon zest and juice, sugar, milk, oil, egg whites, and vanilla extract to the dry ingredients, and stir until the batter is smooth. Using a rubber spatula, gently fold in the figs just until they are evenly distributed throughout the batter.

Pour ¼ cup of the batter into each prepared cup, almost filling it. Bake the muffins on the center rack for 22 minutes, rotating the pan 180 degrees after 15 minutes. When done, the muffins will bounce back slightly when pressed, and a toothpick inserted in the center will come out clean.

Remove the muffins from the oven and let stand for 15 minutes; then transfer to a wire rack, and cool completely. Store the muffins in an airtight container at room temperature for up to 3 days.

Pitta

Cherry Muffins

- 2 cups white whole wheat flour
- 1 teaspoon baking powder
- 1 teaspoon baking soda
- ¼ teaspoon salt
- Zest and juice of 1 lemon
- ⅔ cup raw sugar
- ⅔ cup soy milk
- ½ cup sunflower oil
- 2 egg whites
- 1 tablespoon vanilla extract
- 1 teaspoon almond extract
- 2 cups pitted fresh cherries
- ¼ cup fat-free ricotta cheese

Preheat the oven to 325°F. Line a 12-cup muffin pan with paper liners.

Whisk together the flour, baking powder, baking soda, and salt in a medium bowl. Add the lemon zest and juice, sugar, soy milk, oil, egg whites, vanilla extract, and almond extract to the dry ingredients, and stir until the batter is smooth. Using a rubber spatula, gently swirl in the cherries and the ricotta.

Pour ¼ cup of the batter into each prepared cup, almost filling the cup. Bake the muffins on the center rack for 22 minutes, rotating the pan 180 degrees after 15 minutes. When done, the muffins will bounce back slightly when pressed, and a toothpick inserted in the center will come out clean.

Remove the muffins from the oven and let stand for 15 minutes, then transfer to a wire rack, and cool completely. Store the muffins in an airtight container at room temperature for up to 3 days.

Kapha

Cranberry-Lime Muffins

- 2 cups gluten-free all-purpose baking flour
- 2 teaspoons baking powder
- 2 teaspoons baking soda
- ½ teaspoon salt
- Zest and juice of two limes
- ⅔ cup raw sugar
- ⅔ cup soy milk
- ¼ cup corn oil
- 2 egg whites
- 1 tablespoon vanilla extract
- ½ cup dried cranberries

Preheat the oven to 325°F. Line a 12-cup muffin pan with paper liners.

Whisk together the flour, baking powder, baking soda, and salt in a medium bowl. Add the lime zest and juice, sugar, soy milk, oil, egg whites, and vanilla to the dry ingredients, and stir until the batter is smooth. Using a rubber spatula, gently fold in the cranberries just until they are evenly distributed throughout the batter.

Pour ¼ cup of the batter into each prepared cup, almost filling the cup. Bake the muffins on the center rack for 22 minutes, rotating the pan 180 degrees after 15 minutes. When done, the muffins will bounce back slightly when pressed, and a toothpick inserted in the center will come out clean.

Remove the muffins from the oven and let stand for 15 minutes, then transfer to a wire rack, and cool completely. Store the muffins in an airtight container at room temperature for up to 3 days.

Breakfast Burritos

This is the perfect recipe to use that last handful of veggies left in the crisper. It's also easy to make for one or for a group for brunch. Just preheat the oven and warm the tortillas as soon as guests arrive.

Makes 1 serving

Vata

- 1 whole egg
- 1 egg white
- ½ small jalapeño chili pepper, minced
- ⅛ teaspoon salt
- ⅛ teaspoon freshly ground black pepper
- 1 whole-wheat tortilla (9"), warmed in toaster oven for 1 to 2 minutes
- 4 cherry tomatoes or one small tomato, chopped
- 2 tablespoons reduced-fat mozzarella cheese
- 1 tablespoon basil leaves (3–4 leaves), thinly sliced

Combine the whole egg, egg white, jalapeño pepper, salt, and pepper in a small bowl. Whisk until smooth. Heat a small skillet over medium-high heat. Coat with olive oil cooking spray. Add the egg mixture. Turn once or twice, until the eggs are scrambled and cooked through, about 45 seconds.

Transfer the egg mixture to the center of the tortilla, and top with the tomato, mozzarella, and basil leaves. Wrap, and serve immediately.

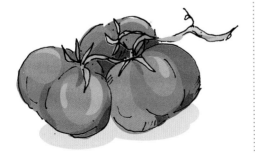

Pitta

- 1 whole egg
- 1 egg white
- ⅛ teaspoon salt
- ⅛ teaspoon freshly ground black pepper
- ¼ cup finely chopped broccoli
- 1 whole-wheat tortilla (9"), warmed in toaster oven for 1 to 2 minutes
- 2 tablespoons goat cheese
- 1 scallion, thinly sliced

Combine the whole egg and egg white, salt, and pepper in a small bowl and set aside. Whisk until smooth. Set aside. Heat a small skillet over medium-high heat. Coat with olive oil cooking spray. Add the broccoli, and cook 4 to 5 minutes, stirring occasionally, until the broccoli is tender-crisp. Add the egg mixture. Turn once or twice, until the eggs are scrambled and cooked through, about 45 seconds.

Transfer the egg mixture to the center of the tortilla, and top with the goat cheese and scallions. Wrap, and serve immediately.

Kapha

- 1 whole egg
- 1 egg white
- ⅛ teaspoon salt
- ⅛ teaspoon freshly ground black pepper
- 2 large mushrooms, stems removed, thinly sliced
- ½ small jalapeño chili pepper, minced
- 1 whole-wheat tortilla (9"), warmed in toaster oven for 1 to 2 minutes

Combine the whole egg and egg white, salt, and pepper in a small bowl. Whisk until smooth. Heat a small skillet over medium-high heat. Coat with olive oil cooking spray. Add the mushrooms and jalapeño pepper. Cook 3 to 4 minutes, stirring occasionally, until the mushrooms are soft. Add the egg mixture. Turn once or twice, until the eggs are scrambled and cooked through, about 45 seconds.

Transfer the egg mixture to the center of the tortilla. Wrap, and serve immediately.

LUNCH AND DINNER

CREAMY VEGETABLE SOUPS

These creamy soups might not seem like they are good for you, but they get their creaminess from light ingredients, such as yogurt (vata), goat cheese (pitta), and soy milk (kapha). Your palate will never know the difference, but your waistline will.

Makes 4 servings

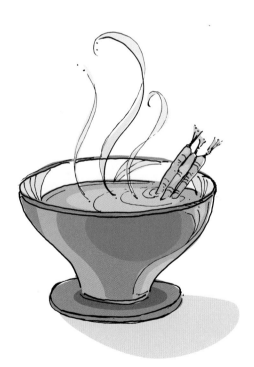

Vata

Cream of Asparagus Soup

1 tablespoon extra-virgin olive oil

1 large bunch of asparagus, ends removed

3 large leeks, white part only, chopped

2 sprigs fresh thyme, leaves only

1 teaspoon lemon zest

¼ teaspoon freshly ground black pepper

¼ teaspoon ground cardamom

⅛ teaspoon ground cloves

½ teaspoon salt

4 cups vegetable or chicken broth

2 cups baby spinach leaves

¼ cup low-fat plain yogurt

Heat the oil in a large stockpot over medium heat. When the oil is warm, add the asparagus. Cook 7 to 10 minutes, until the asparagus starts to brown. Add the leeks, thyme, lemon zest, salt, pepper, cardamom, and cloves. Cook 10 to 15 minutes more, until the leeks soften and the spices become fragrant.

Add the broth, and bring to a boil. Reduce the heat to low, and simmer 10 to 15 minutes. Add the spinach, and cook 2 minutes more, until the spinach has wilted. Add the yogurt. Use an immersion blender to puree directly in the pot, or transfer to a blender in batches to blend. Serve immediately.

Cream of Broccoli Soup

- 1 head of broccoli
- 1 tablespoon extra-virgin olive oil
- 3 large leeks, white part only, chopped
- 1 sprig fresh rosemary, leaves only
- 1 teaspoon fennel seeds
- ½ teaspoon ground cardamom
- 4 cups vegetable or chicken broth
- ½ teaspoon salt
- 3 tablespoons goat cheese

Remove the stalk of the broccoli. Peel the stalk, and cut it into 1″ pieces. Cut the broccoli tops into florets, and set aside. Warm the olive oil in a large stockpot over medium heat. Add the broccoli stalk, leeks, rosemary, fennel seed, and cardamom. Cook 8 to 10 minutes, until the leeks soften and the spices become fragrant.

Add the broth, and bring to a boil. Cover, and cook 10 minutes. Add the reserved broccoli florets and cover, cooking 10 minutes more, until they are soft but still bright green. Add the salt and goat cheese. Use an immersion blender to puree directly in the pot, or transfer to a blender in batches to blend. Serve immediately.

Cream of Broccoli Soup

- 1 head of broccoli
- 1 tablespoon sunflower oil
- 3 large leeks, white part only, chopped
- 2 sprigs fresh thyme, leaves only
- 1 sprig rosemary, leaves only
- ½ teaspoon paprika
- ¼ teaspoon cayenne
- ¼ teaspoon freshly ground black pepper
- 2 cups vegetable or chicken broth
- 2 cups soy milk
- 1 cup cooked navy beans
- ½ teaspoon salt

Remove the stalk of the broccoli. Peel the stalk, and cut into 1″ pieces. Cut the broccoli tops into florets, and set aside. Warm the sunflower oil in a large stockpot over medium heat. Add the broccoli stalks, leeks, thyme, rosemary, paprika, cayenne, and pepper. Cook 8 to 10 minutes, until the leeks soften and the spices become fragrant.

Add the broth and bring to a boil. Cover, and cook 10 minutes, until the broccoli stalks are fork tender. Add the reserved broccoli florets, and cover, cooking 10 minutes more, until they are soft but still bright green. Add the soy milk, beans, and salt. Use an immersion blender to puree directly in the pot, or transfer to a blender in batches to blend. Serve immediately.

Superfood Sandwiches

Sandwiches are a classic American meal. This version cranks up the health using veggies appropriate for your dosha (carrot and onion for vata; avocado, broccoli, and zucchini for pitta; and mushroom, red pepper, and greens for kapha). Take that, corner deli!

Makes 4 servings

Vata

1 tuna steak (about 1 pound), cut into 1" cubes
½ teaspoon salt
¼ teaspoon freshly ground black pepper
2 teaspoons chopped rosemary
Zest and juice of 1 lemon
2 tablespoons extra-virgin olive oil
1 cup pitted black olives, such as kalamata
2 carrots, peeled and shredded
¼ cup parsley leaves, chopped
1 small red onion, minced
2 teaspoons hot sauce, such as Tabasco
½ cup basil leaves, chopped
4 whole wheat pitas
4 large red lettuce leaves

Sprinkle the tuna with the salt, pepper, rosemary, and lemon zest. Heat the oil in a small skillet over medium heat. Add the tuna, and cook 4 to 5 minutes, turning once or twice, until the tuna browns lightly but is still pink in the center.

Meanwhile, combine the olives, lemon juice, carrots, parsley, onion, hot sauce, and basil. Add the tuna, and toss to combine.

Divide the filling among the pitas. Add a lettuce leaf to each one. Serve immediately.

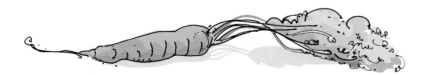

Pitta

- 1 small Hass avocado
- 1 cup broccoli florets
  Zest and juice of 1 lime
- ¼ cup fat-free sour cream
- ½ teaspoon Worcestershire sauce
- ¼ cup chopped red onion
- ½ teaspoon salt
- ¼ teaspoon mild paprika
- 2 baked chicken breasts, cubed
- 1 can (15 ounces) artichoke hearts, rinsed well and drained
- ½ small zucchini, chopped
- 4 whole wheat pitas

Place the avocado, broccoli, lime zest and juice, sour cream, Worcestershire, onion, salt, and paprika in a food processor and pulse to chop. Transfer to a large bowl along with the chicken, artichoke hearts, broccoli, and zucchini. Toss to coat. Fill pitas with the chicken mixture. Serve immediately.

Kapha

- 4 teaspoons corn oil
- 4 large portobello mushroom caps
- 4 cloves garlic, minced
- ¼ cup parsley leaves, chopped
- 1 teaspoon salt
- 1 tablespoon goat cheese
- 1 tablespoon water
- ½ cup roasted red pepper
- 1 cup watercress, chopped, tough stems discarded
- 1 cup spinach
- 4 spelt Roti (page 133)

Heat half of the oil in a large skillet. Add the mushrooms and cook 5 to 6 minutes until the mushrooms soften. Add half of the garlic, half of the parsley, and half of the salt. Cover, and remove from the heat. Set aside.

Place the remaining oil, garlic, parsley, salt, the goat cheese and water in a food processor. Blend until smooth. Toss the red pepper with the watercress and spinach. Spread one roti with one-quarter of the blended spread, top with one-quarter of the mushrooms and one-quarter of the watercress mixture, and fold the roti in half. Repeat to assemble the remaining sandwiches.

Rice and Beans

Rice and beans might not seem like a weight-loss meal, but it is actually very filling—thanks to fiber in the rice and protein in the beans—while being low in calories. Each of these recipes is spiked with the best spices for your dosha.

Makes 4 servings

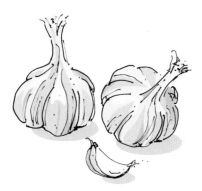

Vata

2 medium sweet potatoes, peeled and cubed

4 teaspoons extra-virgin olive oil

2 teaspoons ground cumin

1 teaspoon salt

½ teaspoon mild chili powder

¼ teaspoon paprika

¼ teaspoon cayenne

1 small onion, chopped

½ green bell pepper, thinly sliced

2 cloves garlic, minced

⅔ cup mung beans, picked through and rinsed

1⅓ cups short-grain brown rice

2½ cups water

½ cup sliced roasted red pepper

2 tablespoons white vinegar

1 tablespoon hot sauce, such as Tabasco

1 tablespoon fresh oregano, minced

¼ teaspoon freshly ground black pepper

Preheat the oven to 400°F. Place the sweet potatoes, half the oil, the cumin, half the salt, chili powder, paprika, and cayenne, in a large bowl. Toss to coat the sweet potatoes. Coat a large baking sheet with cooking spray. Spread the sweet potatoes in an even layer on the baking sheet, and bake 20 to 25 minutes.

Heat the remaining oil in a large skillet. Add the onion, bell pepper, and garlic. Cook 4 to 5 minutes, until the vegetables begin to soften. Add the beans, rice, water, and remaining salt. Cover, and bring to a boil. Reduce the heat to low, and cook 40 to 45 minutes, or until the rice and beans are tender. Stir in red pepper, vinegar, hot sauce, oregano, and black pepper. Stir in the sweet potatoes, and serve immediately.

Pitta

    1 large zucchini, cubed
    2 teaspoons ground cumin
    ½ teaspoon mild chili powder
    ¼ teaspoon paprika
    1 teaspoon salt
    3 teaspoons olive oil
    1 small onion, chopped
    2 cups cauliflower florets
    ½ small jicama, peeled and cubed (about 1 cup)
    ½ green bell pepper, thinly sliced
    1 stalk celery, thinly sliced
    2 cloves garlic, minced
    ⅔ cup mung beans, picked through and rinsed
    1⅓ cups short-grain brown rice
    2½ cups water
    1 tablespoon tomato paste
    1 cup snow peas, cut into 1" pieces
    2 tablespoons white vinegar
    1 tablespoon fresh mint, minced
    ¼ teaspoon freshly ground black pepper

Preheat the oven to 400°F. Place the zucchini, cumin, chili powder, paprika, half the salt, and half the oil in a large bowl. Toss to coat the zucchini. Coat a large baking sheet with cooking spray. Spread the zucchini in an even layer on the baking sheet, and bake 20 to 25 minutes.

Heat the remaining oil in a large skillet. Add the onion, cauliflower, jicama, bell pepper, celery, and garlic. Cook 4 to 5 minutes, until the vegetables begin to soften. Add the beans, rice, water, tomato paste, and remaining salt. Cover, and bring to a boil. Reduce the heat to low, and cook 35 to 40 minutes, or until the rice and beans are almost tender. Add the snow peas, and cook 5 more minutes. Add the vinegar, mint, and black pepper. Stir in the zucchini, and serve immediately.

Kapha

    2 medium sweet potatoes, peeled and cubed
    2 teaspoons ground cumin
    ½ teaspoon chili powder
    ¼ teaspoon paprika
    ¼ teaspoon cayenne
    1 teaspoon salt
    2 to 3 teaspoons safflower oil
    1 small onion, chopped
    ½ green bell pepper, thinly sliced
    2 cloves garlic, minced
    ⅔ cup mung beans, picked through and rinsed
    1⅓ cups pearl barley
    2½ cups water
    ½ cup sliced roasted red pepper
    2 tablespoons white vinegar
      Few dashes of hot sauce, such as Tabasco
    1 tablespoon fresh oregano, minced
    ¼ teaspoon freshly ground black pepper

Preheat the oven to 400°F. Place the sweet potatoes, cumin, chili powder, paprika, cayenne, half the oil, and half the salt in a large bowl. Toss to coat the sweet potatoes. Coat a large baking sheet with cooking spray. Spread the potatoes in an even layer on the baking sheet, and bake 20 to 25 minutes.

Heat the remaining oil in a large skillet. Add the onion, bell pepper, and garlic. Cook 4 to 5 minutes, until the vegetables begin to soften. Add the beans, barley, water, and remaining salt. Cover, and bring to a boil. Reduce the heat to low, and cook 40 to 45 minutes, or until rice and beans are tender. Stir in red pepper, vinegar, hot sauce, oregano, and black pepper. Stir in the sweet potatoes, and serve immediately.

Herbed Risotto

The classic Italian version of this dish usually calls for high-fat mascarpone cheese. However, you can still have creamy risotto without all the fat, if you make it this healthy way, with pureed vegetables and freshly grated Parmesan.

Makes 4 servings

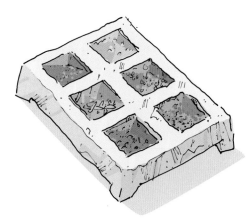

Vata

3 cups low-sodium chicken broth or vegetable broth

1 tablespoon unsalted butter

2 tablespoons extra-virgin olive oil

3 garlic cloves, chopped

2 medium shallots or 1 small yellow onion, chopped very fine

1 cup short-grain brown rice

1 package (10 ounces) frozen squash puree, thawed

¼ cup freshly grated Parmesan cheese

½ teaspoon salt

¼ teaspoon freshly ground black pepper

¼ cup fresh basil leaves, chopped

Bring the broth to a simmer in a medium saucepan over moderately high heat. Reduce the heat to low to keep warm.

Combine the butter and oil in a large saucepan, over moderate heat. Add the garlic and shallots or onion, and cook until softened, about 3 minutes. Add the rice, and cook, stirring, until slightly translucent, about 2 minutes.

Add 1 cup of the warm broth to the rice, and cook over moderately high heat, stirring constantly, until the broth is nearly absorbed. Continue adding the broth, about 1 cup at a time, stirring until it is absorbed before adding more. Simmer uncovered, stirring occasionally. When the rice is cooked through but still firm (about 20 to 25 minutes), add the squash and Parmesan, stirring until the Parmesan is melted. Season with the salt and pepper, and sprinkle with the basil. Serve immediately.

Pitta

- 3 cups low-sodium chicken broth or vegetable broth
- 1 bag (10 ounces) frozen peas, thawed
- ¼ cup water
- 1 tablespoon unsalted butter
- 2 tablespoons extra-virgin olive oil
- 3 garlc cloves, chopped
- 2 medium shallots or 1 small yellow onion, chopped very fine
- 1 cup short-grain brown rice
- ¼ cup freshly grated Parmesan cheese
- ½ teaspoon salt
- ¼ teaspoon freshly ground black pepper
- ¼ cup fresh basil leaves, chopped

Bring the broth to a simmer in a medium saucepan over moderately high heat. Reduce the heat to low to keep warm. Place the peas in a blender with the water, and blend until smooth.

Combine the butter and oil in a large saucepan, over moderate heat. Add the garlic and shallots or onion, and cook until softened, about 3 minutes. Add the rice, and cook, stirring, until slightly translucent, about 2 minutes.

Add 1 cup of the warm broth to the rice, and cook over moderately high heat, stirring constantly, until the broth is nearly absorbed. Continue adding the broth about 1 cup at a time, stirring until it is absorbed before adding more. Simmer uncovered, stirring occasionally. When the rice cooked through but still firm (about 20 to 25 minutes), add the pea puree and Parmesan, stirring until the Parmesan is melted. Season with salt and pepper, and sprinkle with the basil. Serve immediately.

Kapha

- 4 cups low-sodium chicken broth or vegetable broth
- 1 tablespoon corn oil
- 1 tablespoon unsalted butter
- 3 garlc cloves, chopped
- 2 medium shallots or 1 small yellow onion, chopped very fine
- 1 cup pearl barley
- 1 teaspoon hot chili flakes
- 1 bunch of asparagus, trimmed and cut into 1"-pieces
- 2 cups fresh spinach
- ¼ cup freshly grated Parmesan cheese
- ½ teaspoon salt
- ¼ teaspoon freshly ground black pepper
- ¼ cup fresh basil leaves, chopped

Bring the broth to a simmer in a medium saucepan over moderately high heat. Reduce the heat to low to keep warm.

Heat the oil, in a large, deep skillet. Add the butter, garlic, and shallots or onion, and cook over moderate heat, stirring occasionally, until the onion is softened, about 3 minutes. Add the barley and chili flakes. Cook, stirring, for 2 minutes, until the barley is coated in the oil. Add 1 cup of the warm broth, and cook, stirring, until the broth is nearly absorbed. Continue adding the broth, ½ cup at a time, and stirring until it is nearly absorbed before adding more. After about 30 minutes, add the asparagus. Continue adding the broth until the barley is al dente and forms a creamy sauce. Simmer uncovered for about 30 minutes total. Add the asparagus and cook 5 more minutes. Stir in the spinach, and cook an additional minute, until the spinach wilts. Add the Parmesan, and season with the salt and pepper. Sprinkle with the basil, and serve at once, passing more cheese at the table.

Chopped Chicken Salad

Each version of this delicious chicken salad includes the very best fruits, vegetables, and spices for balancing your dosha.

Makes 4 servings

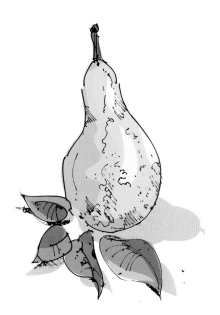

Vata

- 2 boneless, skinless chicken breasts
- ½ teaspoon cumin
- ½ teaspoon salt
- ½ teaspoon freshly ground black pepper
- 2 teaspoons extra-virgin olive oil
- 4 tablespoons raw honey
- 3 tablespoons Dijon mustard
- 2 tablespoons apple cider vinegar
- ¼ teaspoon paprika
- 1 small head romaine lettuce, chopped
- 1 pint cherry tomatoes, cut in half
- 1 small Hass avocado, cubed
- ½ cucumber, peeled and diced
- Kernels of 1 ear corn

Sprinkle the chicken with the cumin, salt, and pepper. Heat the oil in a medium skillet over high heat. Add the chicken, and cook 4 to 5 minutes per side, until the chicken has browned and is cooked through. Set aside.

Whisk the honey, mustard, vinegar, and paprika in a large bowl, until smooth. Add the lettuce, tomatoes, avocado, cucumber, and corn. Cube the reserved chicken, and add it to the vegetable mixture. Toss until well combined. Serve immediately.

Pitta

2 boneless, skinless chicken breasts

½ teaspoon cumin

½ teaspoon salt

½ teaspoon freshly ground black pepper

2 teaspoons extra-virgin olive oil

1 tablespoon raw sugar

1 tablespoon reduced-fat mayonnaise

Zest and juice of 2 limes

2 tablespoons water

½ mango, peeled and diced

1 cup peeled and diced papaya

1 bunch watercress (about 1½ cups), chopped, tough stems discarded

2 stalks celery, thinly sliced

1 small cucumber, peeled and diced (about ¾ cup)

1 small fennel bulb, thinly sliced

Sprinkle the chicken with the cumin, salt, and pepper. Heat the oil in a medium skillet over high heat. Add the chicken, and cook 4 to 5 minutes per side, until the chicken has browned and is cooked through. Set aside.

Whisk the sugar, mayonnaise, lime zest and juice, and water in a large bowl, until smooth. Add the mango, papaya, watercress, celery, cucumber, and fennel. Cube the reserved chicken, and add it to the vegetable mixture. Toss until well combined. Serve immediately.

Kapha

2 boneless, skinless chicken breasts

2 teaspoons curry powder

½ teaspoon salt

½ teaspoon freshly ground black pepper

2 teaspoons corn oil

1 tablespoon raw honey

¼ cup low-fat plain yogurt

Zest and juice of 2 limes

2 tablespoons water

2 heads endive, chopped (about 1 cup)

¼ head broccoli, chopped (about 1 cup)

1 ripe pear, seeded and cubed

2 tablespoons raisins

Sprinkle the chicken with the curry, salt, and pepper. Heat the oil in a medium skillet over high heat. Add the chicken, and cook 4 to 5 minutes per side, until the chicken has browned and is cooked through. Set aside.

Whisk the honey, yogurt, lime zest and juice, and water in a large bowl, until smooth. Add the endive, broccoli, pear, and raisins. Cube the reserved chicken, and add it to the vegetable mixture. Toss until well combined. Serve immediately.

Guacamole and "Chips"

This version of guacamole includes vegetables (tomatoes and corn for vata, spinach and cucumber for pitta, and peas and spinach for kapha) that lower the fat content without losing the luscious taste and creamy texture that we all crave.

Makes 3½ cups

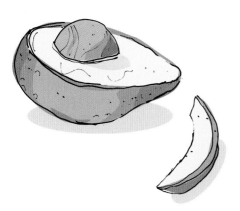

Vata

2 Hass avocados

8 cherry tomatoes, quartered

Kernels of 2 ears corn

½ red onion, chopped

¼ cup cilantro leaves, chopped

1 small jalapeño chili pepper, seeded and diced

Juice of 2 limes

½ teaspoon salt

¼ teaspoon freshly ground black pepper

4 whole wheat pitas, cut into 8 wedges and toasted

Cut the avocados in half, and remove the pits. Scrape the avocado meat into a bowl, and mash it with a fork. Fold in the tomatoes, corn, onion, cilantro, jalapeño pepper, lime juice, salt, and pepper. Serve with the toasted pita chips.

Skinny Suppers

Making lunch the biggest meal of the day while shrinking supper is a key part of *The Yoga Body Diet*. Slimming down dinner is easy to do with this guide. Here, we've taken lunch and dinner recipes that you will find throughout this chapter and provided a version that makes them lighter (lower in fat, calories, and carbohydrates) while still delivering a healthy dose of dosha-balancing superfoods.

Recipe: Creamy Vegetable Soups (page 112)

- These recipes are already Skinny-Supper approved.

Recipe: Chopped Chicken Salad (page 120)

- Use cooking spray instead of olive oil.
- Omit the raw sugar and mayonnaise (pitta) or honey and yogurt (kapha) from the dressing.

Recipe: Dosha Burgers (page 124)

- Use cooking spray instead of oil.
- Skip the pita and the salad; instead, serve the burger on a bed of spinach (cooked for vata; raw for pitta and kapha).

Pitta

- 2 Hass avocados
- 1 cup baby spinach leaves, thinly sliced
- ½ cucumber, peeled, seeded, and diced
- ¼ bulb fennel, diced
- ¼ cup cilantro leaves, chopped
- Juice of 2 limes
- 1 teaspoon ground cumin
- ½ teaspoon salt
- ¼ teaspoon freshly ground black pepper
- 4 whole wheat pitas, cut into 8 wedges and toasted

Cut the avocados in half, and remove the pits. Scrape the avocado meat into a bowl, and mash it with a fork. Fold in the spinach, cucumber, fennel, cilantro, lime juice, cumin, salt, and pepper. Serve with the toasted pita chips.

Kapha

- 1 small jalapeño chili pepper, seeded and cut into 3 pieces
- 1 clove garlic, cut in half
- 3 cups frozen peas, thawed
- 1 cup baby spinach leaves
- 1 tablespoon goat cheese
- 1 teaspoon ground cumin
- Juice of 2 limes
- ¼ cup cilantro leaves, chopped
- ½ teaspoon salt
- ¼ teaspoon freshly ground black pepper
- 4 cups whole grain corn chips

Place the jalapeño pepper and garlic in a food processor, and pulse to chop. Add the peas, spinach, goat cheese, cumin, lime juice, cilantro, salt, and pepper. Puree until smooth. Serve with the chips.

Recipe: Tasty Tacos (page 130)

- Use cooking spray instead of olive oil.
- Eat filling without the tortilla.

Recipe: Tilapia for Your Type (page 136)

- Skip the nut or spice crust. Instead, sprinkle tilapia with a pinch of salt, a pinch of freshly ground black pepper, and the juice of half a lemon. Place the fish in a 7" × 11" baking dish and bake at 400°F for 10 minutes.

Recipe: Vegetable Soufflé (page 140)

- Leave out the cheese.
- Instead of olive oil, use only a squeeze of the fresh lemon or orange.

DOSHA BURGERS

These recipes feature the best proteins for each dosha with a vegetable salad that creates a complete meal.

Makes four 1½-cup servings of salad and four 4-ounce burgers

Vata

Tuna Burgers with Carrot Slaw

Carrot Slaw

- 1 (½") piece ginger, peeled and cut into thirds
- 2 cloves garlic, cut in half
- ¼ teaspoon salt
- 1 tablespoon raw sugar
- ¼ cup reduced-fat mayonnaise
- 1 teaspoon hot chili sauce, such as Sriracha
- 6 large carrots, peeled and grated
- 2 medium beets, peeled and grated

Burgers

- 2 cloves garlic, chopped
- 1 (½") piece ginger, peeled and cut into thirds
- 4 scallions, trimmed and cut into thirds
- ¼ cup cilantro leaves, packed
- 1 pound fresh tuna, cubed
- ½ teaspoon salt
- ½ teaspoon ground star anise (you can do this in a coffee grinder or with a microplane grater)
- 2 egg whites
- ¼ cup rolled oats
- 1 tablespoon sesame oil
- 2 whole wheat pitas, cut in half and warmed

Carrot slaw: Place the ginger, garlic, salt, and sugar in a food processor. Pulse until chopped. Add the mayonnaise and chili sauce.

Pulse until combined. Transfer the mixture to a bowl and stir in beets and carrots until well combined. Set aside.

Burgers: Pulse the garlic and ginger until minced. Add the scallions, cilantro, tuna, salt, and anise. Pulse 3 to 4 times, until a chunky mixture forms. Add the egg whites and oats, pulsing once or twice, until mixed. Form the mixture into 4 equal patties. Heat the oil in a large skillet over medium heat. Add the patties, and cook 4 to 5 minutes per side, until the burgers are cooked through. Slide each burger into a half pita, and serve with the reserved slaw.

Pitta

Chickpea Burgers with Cool Cucumber Salad

Cucumber Salad

- 2 tablespoons reduced-fat mayonnaise
  Zest and juice of 1 lemon
- 1 teaspoon cumin seed, toasted
- 1 teaspoon raw sugar
- ¼ teaspoon salt
- 2 cucumbers, peeled, seeded, and sliced

Burgers

- 2 garlic cloves
- ½ red onion, cut into thirds
- 1 celery stalk, chopped
- 1 cup mushrooms, such as cremini
- ¼ cup flat-leaf parsley, packed
- ¼ cup fresh dill
- 1 can (15 ounces) chick peas, rinsed and drained
- ½ cup rolled oats
  Zest and juice of 1 lemon
- 1 egg white
- 1 teaspoon salt

1 tablespoon extra-virgin olive oil

2 whole-wheat pitas, halved and warmed

2 cups shredded romaine lettuce

Cucumber salad: Place the mayonnaise, lemon zest and juice, cumin seeds, sugar, and salt in a large bowl. Whisk until smooth, and toss with the cucumber slices. Set aside.

Burgers: Place the garlic in a food processor, and pulse until chopped. Add the onion, celery, mushrooms, parsley, and dill, and pulse until finely chopped. Add the chickpeas, oats, egg white, and salt. Pulse 3 to 4 times, until a chunky mixture forms. Form the mixture into 4 equal patties.

Heat the oil in a large skillet over medium heat. Add the patties, and cook 4 to 5 minutes per side, until the burgers are lightly browned and warmed through. Slide each burger into a half pita with one-quarter of the lettuce. Serve burgers with the salad on the side.

Kapha

Black Bean Burgers with Green Bean Salad

Green Bean Salad

1 pound green beans, trimmed and cut into 1"-pieces

¼ cup orange juice

1 tablespoon tomato paste

1 tablespoon corn oil

2 cloves garlic, minced

1 teaspoon fresh thyme leaves

½ teaspoon mild chili powder

½ teaspoon salt

¼ teaspoon freshly ground black pepper

1 red or green bell pepper, diced

½ red onion, minced

Burgers

2 cloves garlic, cut in half

½ red onion, quartered

2 celery stalks, chopped

1 cup mushrooms, such as cremini or white button

1 cup spinach leaves

1 can (15 ounces) black beans, rinsed and drained

½ cup chunky salsa

¼ cup rolled oats

2 egg whites

½ teaspoon salt

¼ teaspoon freshly ground black pepper

1 tablespoon corn oil

2 whole wheat pitas, halved and warmed

Green bean salad: Cover the bottom of a large stockpot with 1" of water. Bring to a boil, and add the green beans. Cook 3 to 4 minutes. Drain through a colander, rinse under cold water, and set aside. In a large bowl, whisk the orange juice, tomato paste, oil, garlic, thyme, chili powder, salt, and black pepper until well combined. Stir in the green beans, bell pepper, and onion. Set aside.

Burgers: Place the garlic in a food processor, and pulse until chopped. Add the onion, celery, mushrooms, spinach, beans, and salsa, and pulse until a chunky mixture forms, 2 to 3 pulses. Add the oats, egg whites, salt, and pepper, pulsing once or twice, until mixed. Form the mixture into 4 equal patties. Heat the oil in a large skillet over medium heat. Add the patties, and cook 4 to 5 minutes per side, until the burgers are lightly browned and warmed through. Slide each burger into a half pita. Serve with the reserved green bean salad.

FRIED RICE

When you cook dishes you love—instead of
bland diet food—you're more likely to be
satisfied and get your fill of healthy foods
such as vegetables, whole grains, and low-fat
proteins. These fried rice recipes are prime
examples of how to do just that.

Makes 4 servings

Vegetable Fried Rice with Peas and Carrots

1 package (14 ounces) extra-firm tofu

1⅓ cups short-grain brown rice

1 tablespoon canola oil

1 (1") piece ginger, peeled and chopped

3 cloves garlic, chopped

2 jalapeño chili peppers, seeded and
   chopped

2 carrots, peeled and chopped

2 cups frozen peas, thawed and rinsed

1 red bell pepper, seeded and thinly sliced

½ teaspoon salt

4 scallions, thinly sliced

Place the tofu in a colander, and place a heavy
pot on top of it. Let the tofu drain for 30
minutes while you cook the rice according to
the package instructions. When the tofu has
given off most of its liquid, dice it, and set
aside.

Heat the oil in a large skillet. Add the ginger,
garlic, and jalapeño peppers, stirring
constantly, 1 to 2 minutes, until the mixture
becomes fragrant. Add the cooked rice,
carrots, peas, and bell pepper and cook 8 to 9
minutes more, until the vegetables start to
soften. Stir in the tofu. Season with the salt
and garnish with the scallions. Serve
immediately.

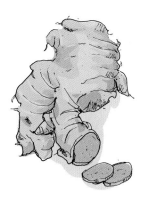

Pineapple Coconut Fried Rice

- 1 package (14 ounces) extra-firm tofu
- 2 cups short-grain brown rice
- 1 tablespoon extra-virgin olive oil
- 1 (1") piece ginger, peeled and chopped
- 3 cloves garlic, chopped
- 2 cups snow peas, cut into thirds
- 2 stalks celery, chopped
- 2 cups green cabbage, thinly sliced
- ½ teaspoon salt
- 1 cup chopped fresh pineapple
- ½ cup toasted unsweetened coconut
- ½ cup fresh cilantro leaves

Place the tofu in a colander, and place a heavy pot on top of it. Let the tofu drain for 30 minutes while you cook the rice according to the package instructions. When the tofu has given off most of its liquid, dice it, and set aside.

Heat the oil in a large skillet. Add the ginger, garlic, snow peas, celery, and cabbage and cook, stirring constantly, 5 minutes, until the mixture becomes fragrant. Add the cooked rice and cook 3 to 4 minutes more, until the vegetables start to soften. Sprinkle with salt. Stir in tofu, pineapple, coconut, and cilantro. Serve immediately.

Szechuan Fried Rice

- 1⅓ cups pearl barley
- 1 tablespoon canola oil
- 1 (1") piece ginger, peeled and chopped
- 3 cloves garlic, chopped
- 1 can (14 ounces) adzuki beans or chick peas, rinsed and drained
- 1 to 2 dried red chili peppers, chopped
- 1 package (10 ounces) shiitake mushrooms, thinly sliced
- 2 cups frozen peas, thawed and rinsed
- 1 red bell pepper, seeded and thinly sliced
- 2 tablespoons apple cider vinegar
- 1 teaspoon raw sugar
- ½ teaspoon salt
- 1 cup baby spinach leaves
- 4 scallions, thinly sliced

Cook the barley according to the package instructions. Heat the oil in a large skillet. Add the ginger and garlic, and cook 1 minute, stirring constantly, until the mixture becomes fragrant. Add the cooked barley, beans, chili peppers, mushrooms, peas, and bell pepper and cook 8 to 9 minutes more, until the vegetables start to soften. Season with the vinegar, sugar, and salt. Add the spinach, and toss until wilted. Garnish with the scallions. Serve immediately.

Pesto Pasta

Pesto pasta makes a refreshing summer meal that can be enjoyed warm or at room temperature. These recipes kick up the flavor and the benefits by adding zucchini and edamame.

Makes 4 servings

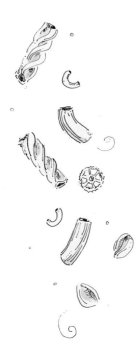

Vata

- 2 cups whole wheat or rice pasta
- 2 medium zucchini
- 1/4 cup pine nuts
- 1 tablespoon extra-virgin olive oil
- 2 cloves garlic
- 2 cups shelled precooked edamame (soy beans)
- 1/2 cup packed fresh basil leaves
- 3/4 teaspoon salt
- 1/4 teaspoon freshly ground black pepper

Cook the pasta according to the package instructions. Reserve 3/4 cup of the cooking liquid before draining. Using a potato peeler, slice the zucchini lengthwise into thick, long ribbons. Set aside.

Heat a medium skillet over medium heat. Add the pine nuts, and toast 4 to 5 minutes, stirring occasionally, until they begin to brown. Remove to a plate. In the same skillet, heat the oil and cook garlic 1 to 2 minutes, until the garlic becomes fragrant but does not brown. Add the zucchini ribbons and 1/4 cup of the reserved pasta water. Simmer the zucchini mixture 2 to 3 minutes, until the zucchini is tender but still bright green.

Blend the pine nuts, edamame, basil, salt, pepper, and remaining pasta water in a blender or food processor, until a smooth paste forms. Place the pasta and the zucchini mixture with its liquid in a large bowl. Toss with the edamame paste until well coated. Serve immediately.

Pitta

- 2 cups whole wheat or rice pasta
- 2 medium zucchini
- ¼ cup pine nuts
- 1 tablespoon extra-virgin olive oil
- ½ teaspoon ground cumin
- 2 cups shelled precooked edamame
- ¼ cup packed fresh basil leaves
- 1 teaspoon salt

Cook the pasta according to the package instructions. Reserve ¾ cup of the cooking liquid before draining. Using a potato peeler or vegetable slicer, slice the zucchini lengthwise into thick, long ribbons. Set aside.

Heat a medium skillet over medium heat. Add the pine nuts, and toast 4 to 5 minutes, stirring occasionally, until they begin to brown. Remove to a plate. In the same skillet, heat the oil and cumin for 1 minute, until the cumin becomes fragrant. Add the reserved zucchini ribbons and ¼ cup of the reserved pasta water. Let the zucchini simmer 2 to 3 minutes, until it is tender but still bright green. Set aside.

Blend the pine nuts, edamame, basil, salt, and the remaining pasta water in a blender or food processor until a smooth paste forms. Place the cooked pasta and the zucchini mixture with its liquid in a large bowl. Toss with the edamame paste until well coated. Serve immediately.

Kapha

- 2 cups whole-grain corn spaghetti or other corn pasta (available at health food stores)
- 2 medium zucchini (about 1 pound)
- ¼ cup pine nuts
- 1 tablespoon extra-virgin olive oil
- 2 cloves garlic
- 2 cups shelled pre-cooked edamame
- ¼ cup packed fresh basil leaves
- 1 teaspoon salt
- ¼ teaspoon freshly ground black pepper

Cook the pasta according to the package instructions. Reserve ¾ cup of the cooking liquid before draining. Using a potato peeler, slice the zucchini lengthwise into thick, long ribbons. Set aside.

Heat a medium skillet over medium heat. Add the pine nuts, and toast 4 to 5 minutes, stirring occasionally, until they begin to brown. Remove to a plate. In the same skillet, heat the oil and cook the garlic for 1 to 2 minutes, until it becomes fragrant but does not brown. Add the reserved zucchini ribbons and ¼ cup of the reserved pasta water. Let the zucchini simmer 2 to 3 minutes, until it is tender but still bright green. Set aside.

Blend the pine nuts, edamame, basil, salt, pepper, and the remaining pasta water in a blender or food processor. Blend until a smooth paste forms. Place the pasta and the zucchini mixture with its liquid in a large bowl. Toss with the edamame paste until well coated. Serve immediately.

Tasty Tacos

Mexican food can be healthy when it's made with delicious, high-quality ingredients. Using fish instead of beef provides a wonderful source of lean protein and heart-healthy omega-3 fatty acids. Vata will benefit from salmon, which is rich, heavy, and oily; while pitta and kapha will enjoy tilapia, which is light and flaky.

Makes 4 servings

Vata

- 1 tablespoon extra-virgin olive oil
- 2 large yellow onions, thinly sliced
- 1 teaspoon raw sugar
- ½ teaspoon salt
- 12 ounces wild salmon, skin removed, cut into 1" slices
- ½ teaspoon saffron threads
- ½ teaspoon ground turmeric
- 1 pint brussels sprouts, chopped
- 8 fajita-sized whole wheat tortillas, warmed
- 1 cup mild salsa

Heat the oil in a large skillet over high heat. Add the onions, sugar, and salt, stirring once. Cook 1 to 2 minutes, until the onions start to brown, then reduce the heat to medium, and continue to cook 15 to 20 minutes, until the onions are golden brown.

Sprinkle the salmon with the saffron and turmeric. Add it to the skillet, and increase the heat to medium-high. Cook the salmon 4 to 5 minutes, turning once, until the salmon starts to cook on the outside. Add the brussels sprouts, cover, and cook for 1 minute. Divide the salmon mixture among the 8 tortillas, and top each with a tablespoon of the salsa. Serve immediately.

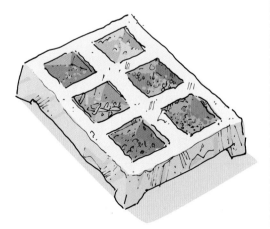

Pitta

Pico de Gallo

3 ripe plum tomatoes (about ¾ pound), quartered

½ small red or yellow onion

½ small jicama, peeled and cut into chunks

1 clove garlic, minced

2 teaspoons fresh lime juice

¼ teaspoon salt

¼ cup cilantro, chopped

Tacos

12 ounces tilapia fillets

½ teaspoon salt

½ teaspoon ground cumin

½ teaspoon mild chili powder

¼ teaspoon ground coriander

1 tablespoon extra-virgin olive oil

8 fajita-sized whole wheat tortillas, warmed

½ red or green cabbage, thinly sliced

1 cup sprouts, such as alfalfa or broccoli

In the bowl of a food processor, combine all the ingredients for the pico de gallo, and pulse until the salsa is slightly chunky, about 7 pulses.

Sprinkle the tilapia with the salt, cumin, chili powder, and coriander. Heat the oil in a large skillet over high heat. Add the fish, and cook 4 to 5 minutes per side, turning once. Break the fish into chunks.

Divide the pico de gallo among the tortillas, and top with the fish. Sprinkle with the cabbage and sprouts, and serve immediately.

Kapha

Chipotle Salsa

1 pint cherry or grape tomatoes

3 cloves garlic, skins intact

½ small red or yellow onion

1 chipotle chili pepper in adobo sauce

1 tablespoon adobo sauce from jar of chipotle chile peppers

2 teaspoons fresh lime juice

¼ cup cilantro, chopped

¼ teaspoon salt

Tacos

12 ounces tilapia fillets

½ teaspoon salt

1 tablespoon extra-virgin olive oil

½ red or green cabbage, thinly sliced

8 corn tortillas, warmed

4 radishes, thinly sliced

1 cup sprouts, such as alfalfa or broccoli

To make the salsa: Heat a large dry skillet over high heat. Add the tomatoes and garlic, and cook 4 to 5 minutes, until the garlic skins start to blacken. Carefully peel the garlic and place it in a food processor along with the onion, tomatoes, chipotle pepper, adobo sauce, lime juice, cilantro, and salt. Pulse until the salsa is slightly chunky, about 7 pulses.

Sprinkle the tilapia with the salt. Heat the oil in a large skillet over high heat. Add the fish, and cook 4 to 5 minutes per side, turning once. Break the fish into chunks.

Divide the salsa among the tortillas, and top with the fish. Sprinkle with the cabbage, radishes, and sprouts, and serve immediately.

Roti Pizza

Roti is a light, sweet-tasting flatbread. It's an Indian staple. We've combined it with savory pizza ingredients. Each recipe keeps fat and calories in check by using fresh, whole food ingredients like baby spinach, garlic, and basil.

Makes 4 servings

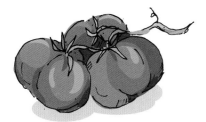

Vata

Roti

2½ cups whole wheat flour
½ teaspoon salt
1 cup warm water

Toppings

4 tablespoons tomato paste
2 cloves garlic, minced
4 large tomatoes, thinly sliced
2 cups baby spinach leaves, chopped
2 cups shredded reduced-fat mozzarella cheese
½ cup fresh basil leaves, thinly sliced

Preheat the oven to 400°F. Place 2 cups of the flour in a food processor with the salt. Pulse while adding the water gradually, until a soft, sticky dough begins to form. Place the dough in a bowl, and continue to knead it, using additional flour to keep it from sticking to your fingers. Separate the dough into 4 evenly-sized pieces. Roll each piece into a ball. Place on the countertop, and cover with a dish towel. Let it rest for 10 minutes.

Roll out each piece of dough into a 8″-round about ⅛″-thick. Rub each piece with 1 tablespoon of the tomato paste. Top with the garlic, tomatoes, spinach, and mozzarella. Bake 10 to 15 minutes on a baking sheet, until the dough is cooked through and the cheese is bubbly. Sprinkle with the basil, and serve immediately.

Pitta

Roti

2½ cups whole wheat flour
½ teaspoon salt
1 cup warm water

Toppings

4 tablespoons tomato paste
2 cloves garlic, minced
1 small bunch asparagus, cut into
   1"-pieces
1 can (15 ounces) quartered artichoke
   hearts, rinsed well and drained
2 cups cherry tomatoes, cut in half
2 cups shredded reduced-fat mozzarella
   cheese
½ cup fresh basil leaves, thinly sliced

Preheat the oven to 400°F. Place 2 cups of the flour in a food processor with the salt. Pulse while adding the water gradually, until a soft, sticky dough begins to form. Place the dough in a bowl, and continue to knead it, using additional flour to keep it from sticking to your fingers. Separate the dough into 4 evenly-sized pieces. Roll each piece into a ball. Place on the countertop, and cover with a dish towel. Let is rest for 10 minutes.

Roll out each piece of dough into a 8″-round about ⅛″-thick. Rub each piece with 1 tablespoon of the tomato paste. Top with the garlic, asparagus, artichokes, tomatoes, and mozzarella. Bake 10 to 15 minutes on a baking sheet, until the dough is cooked through and the cheese is bubbly. Sprinkle with the basil, and serve immediately.

Kapha

Roti

2¾ cups spelt flour (available at
   health food stores)
½ teaspoon salt
1 cup warm water

Toppings

4 tablespoons tomato paste
2 cloves garlic, minced
1 red bell pepper, thinly sliced
2 cups baby spinach, chopped
2 cups shredded reduced-fat mozzarella
   cheese
½ cup fresh basil leaves, thinly sliced

Preheat the oven to 400°F. Place 2½ cups of the flour in a food processor with the salt. Pulse while adding the water gradually, until a soft, sticky dough begins to form. Place the dough in a bowl, and continue to knead it, using additional flour to keep it from sticking to your fingers. Separate the dough into 4 evenly-sized pieces. Roll each piece into a ball. Place on the countertop, and cover with a dish towel. Let it rest for 10 minutes.

Roll out each piece of dough into an 8″-round about ⅛″-thick. Rub each piece with 1 tablespoon of the tomato paste. Top with the garlic, bell pepper, spinach, and mozzarella. Bake 10 to 15 minutes on a baking sheet, until the dough is cooked through and the cheese is bubbly. Sprinkle with the basil, and serve immediately.

FISH IN PHYLLO

Even if you've never cooked fish, this light, flaky dish is easy. The phyllo keeps the fish from drying out and makes a crisp packet that can satisfy cravings for crunchy foods. Each recipe includes an ideal veggie for your dosha.

Makes 4 servings

Vata

Trout in Phyllo Packet with Shaved Brussels Sprouts

Zest and juice of 1 small lemon
1 tablespoon Dijon mustard
¼ teaspoon freshly ground black pepper
¼ teaspoon ground cardamom
1 teaspoon raw sugar
4 trout fillets (4 ounces each)
¾ teaspoon salt
4 phyllo pastry sheets
4 scallions, thinly sliced
1 carrot, grated
1 tablespoon extra-virgin olive oil
4 cloves garlic, minced
4 large tomatoes, diced
1 (1") piece ginger, peeled and grated

Preheat the oven to 350°F. Mix the lemon juice (reserve the zest), mustard, pepper, cardamom, and sugar in a small bowl. Sprinkle the 4 fillets with ½ teaspoon of the salt, and top with the lemon mixture. Coat one sheet of the phyllo dough with a light layer of olive oil cooking spray. Fold in half. Set a piece of the fish in the center, and sprinkle with one-quarter each of the scallions and carrot. Fold the phyllo dough as if folding a shirt and transfer seam-side down to a baking sheet with a spatula. Repeat with remaining phyllo sheets and fillets. Coat the top of the phyllo packets with a light layer of cooking spray, and bake 15 to 20 minutes, until the tops are lightly browned.

Heat the olive oil in a small saucepan over medium-high heat while the fish is baking. Add the garlic, and cook 1 to 2 minutes, until the garlic lightly browns. Add the tomatoes and the remaining salt, cooking an additional 4 to 5 minutes, until most of the liquid evaporates and the tomatoes soften. Stir in the ginger and reserved lemon zest. Divide the tomato sauce evenly among 4 soup bowls or plates. Top with a phyllo packet, and serve immediately.

Pitta

Trout in Phyllo Packet with Shaved Asparagus

½ pound asparagus, trimmed
Zest and juice of 1 small lemon
1 tablespoon reduced-fat mayonnaise
2 tablespoons cilantro leaves, chopped
¼ teaspoon freshly ground black pepper
¼ teaspoon ground cardamom
1 teaspoon raw sugar
4 trout fillets (4 ounces each)
¾ teaspoon salt
4 phyllo pastry sheets
1 tablespoon extra-virgin olive oil
½ bulb fennel, chopped
2 cloves garlic, chopped
2 large tomatoes, diced
1 (1") piece ginger, peeled and grated

Preheat the oven to 350°F. Using a potato peeler, shave the asparagus into thin strips. Coarsely chop any remaining ends, and set aside. Mix the lemon juice (reserve the zest), mayonnaise, cilantro, pepper, cardamom, and sugar in a small bowl. Sprinkle the 4 fillets with $\frac{1}{2}$ teaspoon of the salt, and rub with the mayonnaise mixture. Coat one sheet of the phyllo dough with a light layer of olive oil cooking spray. Fold in half. Set a piece of the fish in the center, and sprinkle with one-quarter of the reserved asparagus. Fold the phyllo dough as if folding a shirt and transfer seam-side down to a baking sheet with a spatula. Repeat with the remaining phyllo sheets and fillets. Coat the top of the phyllo packets with a light layer of cooking spray, and bake 15 to 20 minutes, until the tops are lightly browned.

Heat the olive oil in a small saucepan over medium-high heat while the fish is baking. Add the fennel and garlic, and cook 4 to 5 minutes, until the fennel softens and the garlic lightly browns. Add the tomatoes and the remaining salt, cooking an additional 4 to 5 minutes, until most of the liquid evaporates and the tomatoes soften. Stir in the ginger and reserved lemon zest. Divide the tomato sauce evenly among 4 soup bowls or plates. Top with a phyllo packet, and serve immediately.

Kapha

Trout in Phyllo Packet with Baby Spinach

3 cloves garlic, minced

1 tablespoon spicy mustard

$\frac{1}{4}$ teaspoon freshly ground black pepper

$\frac{1}{4}$ teaspoon ground cayenne

1 teaspoon raw sugar

1 teaspoon chopped thyme leaves

4 trout fillets (4 ounces each)

$\frac{3}{4}$ teaspoon salt

4 phyllo pastry sheets

2 cups baby spinach, chopped

1 tablespoon extra-virgin olive oil

4 cloves garlic, minced

1 small jalapeño chili pepper, seeded and chopped

4 large tomatoes, diced

1 (1") piece ginger, peeled and grated

Preheat oven to 350°F. Mix the garlic, mustard, pepper, cayenne, sugar, and thyme in a small bowl. Sprinkle the 4 fillets with $\frac{1}{2}$ teaspoon of the salt and rub with the mustard mixture. Coat one sheet of the phyllo dough with a light layer of olive oil cooking spray. Fold in half. Set a piece of the fish in the center and sprinkle with one-fourth of the baby spinach. Fold the phyllo dough as if folding a shirt and transfer seam-side down to a baking sheet with a spatula. Repeat with remaining phyllo sheets and fillets. Coat the top of the phyllo packets with a light layer of cooking spray, and bake 15 to 20 minutes until, the tops arelightly browned.

Heat the olive oil in a small saucepan over medium-high heat while the fish is baking. Add the garlic, and cook 1 to 2 minutes, until the garlic lightly browns. Add the jalapeño pepper, tomatoes, and the remaining salt, cooking an additional 4 to 5 minutes, until most of the liquid evaporates and the tomatoes soften. Stir in the ginger. Divide the tomato sauce evenly among 4 soup bowls or plates. Top with a phyllo packet, and serve immediately.

TILAPIA FOR YOUR TYPE

Fish crusted in nuts or spices might sound like a fancy restaurant dish, but you can enjoy it at home, the healthy way. Nuts are high in monounsaturated fatty acids that offer a slew of benefits, including improving heart health and preventing disease.

Makes 4 servings

Vata

Hazelnut-Crusted Tilapia with Mashed Sweet Potatoes and Carrots

Mashed Sweet Potatoes

- 3 medium sweet potatoes (about 1 pound)
- 2 carrots, peeled and grated
  Zest and juice of 1 orange
- 1 tablespoon ghee (page 101)
- ½ teaspoon salt
- ¼ teaspoon cinnamon

Tilapia

- 2 tablespoons whole wheat flour
- ½ cup hazelnuts, finely chopped
- 1 cup cooked quinoa
- 2 egg whites
- 4 tilapia fillets (6 ounces each)
- ½ teaspoon salt
- ¼ teaspoon freshly ground black pepper
- 1 tablespoon extra-virgin olive oil

Preheat the oven to 400°F. Poke the potatoes with a fork and place in a baking dish. Bake 45 to 50 minutes, until the potatoes are soft to the touch. (Leave the oven at the same temperature to cook the fish.) Place the carrots and orange juice (reserve the zest) in a small saucepan, and warm over medium heat for 4 to 5 minutes, until the carrots begin to soften. Scoop the potato flesh out of the peels and into a large bowl. Add the carrot mixture, ghee, salt, and cinnamon. Mash with a fork until well combined, and set aside until ready to serve.

Mix the flour and reserved orange zest in a shallow dish. Mix the nuts and quinoa together, and spread on a piece of wax paper. Beat the egg whites, and pour into a shallow plate or bowl. Sprinkle the fish with the salt and pepper. Turn each fillet in the flour mixture, then in egg whites, then press each side into the nut mixture.

Preheat a large skillet over medium-high heat. Add the oil, then the fish fillets, browning 2 minutes on each side. Transfer to a baking dish. Bake 8 to 10 minutes, until the fish flakes when pressed with a fork. Serve immediately with the mashed sweet potatoes.

Pitta

Coriander-Crusted Tilapia with Broccoli

- 2 tablespoons whole wheat flour
  Zest and juice of 1 lemon
- 1 cup cooked quinoa
- ½ cup almonds, chopped fine
- 1 tablespoon coriander seeds, crushed with a heavy skillet
- 2 large egg whites
- 4 tilapia fillets (6 ounces each)
- ½ teaspoon salt

1 tablespoon extra-virgin olive oil

4 garlic cloves, minced

2 small heads broccoli, cut into florets

½ cup chicken or vegetable broth

8 scallions, chopped

Preheat the oven to 400°F. To make the crust: Place the flour and lemon zest in a shallow dish. Mix the quinoa, almonds, and crushed coriander together and spread on a piece of waxed paper. Beat egg whites and pour into a shallow plate or bowl. Sprinkle the fish with salt. Turn each fillet in the flour mixture, then in egg whites, then press each side into nut mixture.

Heat a large skillet over medium-high heat. Add the oil, then the fish fillets, browning 2 minutes on each side. Transfer to a baking dish. Bake 8 to 10 minutes, until the fish flakes when pressed with a fork.

While the fish is baking, heat another large skillet over medium-high heat. Add the garlic and broccoli, and cook 3 to 4 minutes, until the garlic becomes fragrant. Add the broth and the lemon juice, and cover. Cook 4 to 5 minutes more, until most of the broth has evaporated and the broccoli is tender-crisp. Top with the scallions, and serve immediately with the fish.

Cajun-Style Herb-Crusted Tilapia with Garlicky Green Beans

1 pound green beans, trimmed and cut into thirds

Kernels of 2 ears corn (about 1 cup)

Zest and juice of 1 lemon

2 tablespoons corn oil

3 cloves garlic, minced

2 teaspoons Dijon mustard

2 teaspoons granulated raw sugar

¼ cup fresh cilantro or parsley

½ cup corn flour

2 teaspoons paprika

1 teaspoon chopped fresh oregano leaves

1 teaspoon chopped fresh thyme leaves

½ teaspoon cayenne

½ teaspoon freshly ground black pepper

½ tablespoon ground coriander

4 tilapia fillets (6 ounces each)

½ teaspoon salt

Preheat the oven to 400°F. Cover the bottom of a large stockpot with 1″ of water. Bring to a boil, and add the green beans. Cover and cook 4 to 5 minutes, until the beans are tender-crisp. Drain, and transfer to a large bowl. Toss with the corn kernels, lemon zest and juice, half of the oil, and the garlic, mustard, sugar, and cilantro or parsley. Set aside.

Mix the corn flour with the paprika, oregano, thyme, cayenne, black pepper, and coriander and spread onto a plate. Sprinkle the fish with half of the saltm and press both sides of each fillet into the flour mixture. Heat the remaining oil in a large ovenproof skillet over high heat. Add the fish fillets and cook 2 to 3 minutes, until the coating begins to brown. Turn them and slide the skillet into the oven. Bake 7 to 9 minutes, until the fish flakes with a fork. Serve immediately with the green beans.

CHICKEN QUESADILLAS

Quesadillas aren't just for snacks or football games. You can turn yours into a quick-to-prepare weeknight meal. Using whole grain tortillas makes them naturally lower in simple carbohydrates.

Makes 4 servings

Vata

Chicken Quesadillas with Fresh Jalapeño-Tomato Salsa

Salsa

- 2 medium tomatoes, diced
  Juice of 2 limes
- ¼ cup packed cilantro leaves, thinly sliced
- 1 jalapeño chili pepper, seeded, finely chopped
- ¼ teaspoon salt

Quesadillas

- 4 boneless, skinless chicken breasts, thinly sliced
- 1 teaspoon salt
- 1 teaspoon ground cumin
- 1 teaspoon mild chili powder
- 8 whole wheat tortillas (9")
- 2 cups baby spinach leaves
- ½ cup grated reduced-fat mozzarella cheese

Combine the tomatoes, lime juice, cilantro, jalapeño pepper, and salt. Stir until well combined, and set aside.

Preheat the oven to 400°F. Cover two baking sheets with aluminum foil, and coat them with cooking spray. Sprinkle the chicken with salt, cumin, and chili powder, and place it on the baking sheets. Bake 10 to 12 minutes, until the chicken is cooked through and no longer pink in the center. Transfer the chicken with the foil onto a heatproof countertop.

Coat the same two baking sheets with cooking spray. Place 2 tortillas on each sheet. Top each with one-quarter of the chicken slices, one-quarter of the spinach, and 2 tablespoons of the cheese. Cover with one of the remaining tortillas. Coat again with a light layer of cooking spray. Bake 10 to 15 minutes, until the cheese is melted and the tortillas begin to brown lightly. Serve immediately with the reserved salsa.

Pitta

Chicken-Zucchini Quesadillas with Cilantro-Mango Salsa

Salsa

- 1 mango, peeled and cubed
- ½ small cucumber, peeled and cubed
  Juice of 2 limes
- ¼ cup packed cilantro leaves, thinly sliced
- ¼ teaspoon salt

Quesadillas

- 4 boneless, skinless chicken breasts, thinly sliced
- 1 teaspoon salt
- 1 teaspoon ground cumin
- 1 teaspoon ground coriander
- 8 whole wheat tortillas (9")
- 1 small zucchini, thinly sliced
- ½ cup grated reduced-fat mozzarella cheese

Combine the mango, cucumber, lime juice, cilantro, and salt. Stir until well combined, and set aside.

Preheat the oven to 400°F. Cover two baking sheets with aluminum foil, and coat them with cooking spray. Sprinkle the chicken with the salt, cumin, and coriander, and place it on the baking sheets. Bake 10 to 12 minutes, until the chicken is cooked through and no longer pink in the center. Transfer the chicken with the foil onto a heatproof countertop.

Coat the same two baking sheets with cooking spray. Place 2 tortillas on each sheet. Top each with one-quarter of the chicken slices, one-quarter of the zucchini, and 2 tablespoons of the cheese. Cover with one of the remaining tortillas. Coat again with a light layer of cooking spray. Bake 10 to 15 minutes, until the cheese is melted and the tortillas begin to brown lightly. Serve immediately with the reserved salsa.

Kapha

Chicken-Mushroom Quesadillas with Chipotle-Lime Corn Salsa

Salsa

    1 medium tomato, diced
       Kernels of 2 ears corn (about 1 cup)
       Juice of 2 limes
    ¼ cup packed cilantro leaves, thinly sliced
    1 small chipotle chili pepper in adobo sauce, chopped
    1 tablespoon adobo sauce from jar of chipotle chilies
    ¼ teaspoon salt

Quesadillas

    4 boneless, skinless chicken breasts, sliced thinly
    1 teaspoon salt
    1 teaspoon ground cumin
    ¼ teaspoon cayenne
    ¼ teaspoon freshly ground black pepper
    8 gluten-free tortillas (9")
    1 red bell pepper, thinly sliced
    2 cups white mushrooms, thinly sliced
    ½ cup fat-free ricotta cheese

Combine the tomato, corn, lime juice, chipotle pepper, cilantro, adobo sauce, and salt. Stir until well combined, and set aside.

Preheat the oven to 400°F. Cover two baking sheets with aluminum foil, and coat them with cooking spray. Sprinkle the chicken with salt, cumin, cayenne, and black pepper, and place it on the baking sheets. Bake 10 to 12 minutes, until the chicken is cooked through and no longer pink in the center. Transfer the chicken with the foil onto a heatproof countertop.

Coat the same two baking sheets with cooking spray. Place 2 tortillas on each sheet. Top each with one-quarter of the chicken slices, one-quarter each of the bell pepper and mushrooms, and 2 tablespoons of the ricotta. Cover with one of the remaining tortillas. Coat again with a light layer of cooking spray. Bake 10 to 15 minutes, until the cheese is warmed through and the tortillas begin to brown lightly. Serve immediately with the reserved salsa.

VEGETABLE SOUFFLÉ

You don't have to be a chef to make these luscious soufflés, which puff up beautifully without your whipping egg whites all evening. They are perfect for Mother's Day or an elegant brunch or simply a rainy evening when a plain salad just won't do.

Makes 4 servings

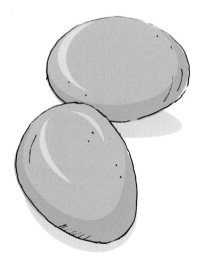

Tomato-Garlic Soufflé with Spinach Salad

- 2 cloves garlic, thinly sliced
- 2 large tomatoes, chopped
- 2 whole eggs
- 4 egg whites
- 2 tablespoons goat cheese
- 2 tablespoons whole wheat flour
- ½ teaspoon baking powder
- ¼ teaspoon salt
- 4 cups baby spinach leaves
- 2 lemons, cut into wedges
- 2 teaspoons extra-virgin olive oil

Preheat the oven to 400° F. Coat four ½-cup ramekins or oven-safe coffee mugs with cooking spray. Heat a small skillet over high heat. Coat with cooking spray, and add the garlic, cooking 1 to 2 minutes, until the garlic becomes fragrant. Add the tomatoes, and cook an additional 1 to 2 minutes, until most of the liquid is evaporated. Set the skillet aside to cool slightly.

In a large bowl, combine the whole eggs, egg whites, goat cheese, flour, baking powder, and salt. Add the tomato mixture, and combine well. Divide the egg mixture among 4 ramekins, and bake 12 to 14 minutes, until the soufflés are puffed and no longer runny in the center.

Divide the spinach among 4 plates. Drizzle with the lemon, and drizzle with the olive oil. Serve immediately with the soufflés.

Pitta

Zucchini Soufflé with Watercress Salad

    1   large zucchini, thinly sliced
    1/2 teaspoon salt
    2   whole eggs
    4   egg whites
    1/4 cup packed cilantro leaves
    2   tablespoons reduced-fat goat cheese
    2   tablespoons whole wheat flour
    1/2 teaspoon baking powder
    1/4 teaspoon salt
    2   bunches watercress (about 3 cups),
        rinsed and chopped, tough stems
        discarded
    1   small orange, quartered
    2   teaspoons extra-virgin olive oil

Preheat the oven to 400° F. Coat four 1/2-cup ramekins or oven-safe coffee mugs with cooking spray. Heat a small skillet over high heat. Coat with cooking spray, add the zucchini, and reduce to medium heat. Cook 3 to 4 minutes, until the zucchini starts to brown. Set the skillet aside to cool slightly.

In a large bowl, combine the whole eggs, egg whites, cilantro, goat cheese, flour, baking powder, salt, and zucchini, and mix until well combined. Divide the egg mixture among 4 ramekins, and bake 12 to 14 minutes, until the soufflés are puffed and no longer runny in the center.

Divide the watercress among 4 plates. Drizzle with the orange, and drizzle with the olive oil. Serve immediately with the soufflés.

Kapha

Asparagus Soufflé with Baby Spinach Salad

    1/2 pound asparagus (about 8 spears),
        thinly sliced
    1/2 green bell pepper, diced
    2   cloves garlic, thinly sliced
    2   whole eggs
    4   egg whites
    2   tablespoons reduced-fat goat cheese
    2   tablespoons amaranth flour or oat flour
    1/2 teaspoon baking powder
    1/4 teaspoon salt
    4   cups baby spinach leaves
    2   lemons, cut into wedges
    2   teaspoons extra-virgin olive oil

Preheat the oven to 400° F. Coat four 1/2-cup ramekins or oven-safe coffee mugs with cooking spray. Heat a medium skillet over high heat. Coat with cooking spray, and add the asparagus, bell pepper, and garlic. Reduce the heat to medium, and cook 3 to 4 minutes, until the garlic becomes fragrant. Set the skillet aside to cool slightly.

In a large bowl, combine the whole eggs, egg whites, goat cheese, flour, baking powder, and salt. Add the asparagus mixture and mix until well combined. Divide the egg mixture among 4 ramekins, and bake 13 to 15 minutes, until the soufflés are puffed and no longer runny in the center.

Divide the spinach among 4 plates. Drizzle with the lemon, and drizzle with the olive oil. Serve immediately with the soufflés.

Tea-Poached Chicken with Vegetables

Tea gives the chicken an attractive caramel-brown color and infuses it with subtle flavor, adding to a dish that is packed with protein and dosha-friendly tender vegetables.

Makes 4 servings

Vata

    4   tea bags, such as Darjeeling
    1   pod star anise
    1   cinnamon stick
    1   teaspoon black peppercorns
    1   medium orange, with peel
    ¼   teaspoon salt
    4   boneless, skinless chicken breasts
    1   tablespoon peanut butter or almond butter
    4   cloves garlic, minced
    2   teaspoons hot chili sauce, such as Sriracha
    2   teaspoons sesame seeds
    2   teaspoons ground flaxseeds
    1   tablespoon sesame oil
    2   carrots, thinly sliced
    1   red bell pepper, seeded and thinly sliced
    1   red onion, cubed
    2   cups snow peas, cut into thirds
    4   cups baby spinach leaves

Bring 8 cups of water to a boil in a medium saucepan. Add the tea, anise, cinnamon, peppercorns, and a 2″ strip of orange peel. Cover, turn off the heat, and steep for 10 minutes. Squeeze and discard the tea bags. Return the tea to a slow boil. Add the chicken, and cook 5 minutes. Cover the pan, and remove it from the heat. Let it stand 30 minutes or until the chicken is cooked through. Remove the chicken from pot and let it cool to room temperature. Slice the chicken into long, thin pieces. Set aside.

Meanwhile, squeeze the juice from the orange into a small bowl. Add the peanut butter or almond butter, garlic, and chili sauce. Whisk until smooth, and set aside. Heat a large dry skillet over medium heat. Add the sesame seeds and flaxseeds. Cook 2 to 3 minutes, stirring constantly, until the seeds are fragrant and toasted. Transfer to a plate. Add the sesame oil to the skillet. Add the carrots, bell pepper, onion, and snow peas. Cook 5 to 6 minutes, until the vegetables start to soften. Add the spinach and the reserved orange juice mixture, and reduce the heat to low. Cook 1 to 2 minutes more until the sauce thickens and the spinach wilts. Arrange the reserved chicken on a serving plate, top with the vegetables and sauce, and sprinkle with the reserved sesame seeds and flaxseeds. Serve immediately.

Pitta

    4   tea bags, such as Darjeeling or Chinese oolong
    1   pod star anise
    1   cinnamon stick
    1   medium orange, with peel
    4   boneless, skinless chicken breasts
    1   tablespoon almond butter
    4   cloves garlic, minced
    2   teaspoons tomato paste
    1   tablespoon extra-virgin olive oil
    2   carrots, thinly sliced
    1   pound asparagus, trimmed and cut into 1″-pieces
    1   red onion, cubed
    2   cups snow peas, cut into thirds

2 cups broccoli florets
4 teaspoons ground flaxseeds

Bring 8 cups of water to a boil in a medium saucepan. Add the tea, anise, cinnamon, peppercorns, and a 2″-strip of orange peel. Cover, turn off the heat, and steep for 10 minutes. Squeeze and discard the tea bags. Return the tea to a slow boil. Add the chicken, and cook 5 minutes. Cover the pan, and remove it from the heat. Let it stand 30 minutes or until the chicken is cooked through. Remove the chicken from the pot and let it cool to room temperature. Slice the chicken into long, thin pieces. Set aside.

Meanwhile, squeeze the juice from the orange into a small bowl. Add the almond butter, garlic, and tomato paste. Whisk until smooth, and set aside. Heat the oil in a large skillet over medium-high heat. Add the carrots, asparagus, onion, snow peas, and broccoli. Cook 5 to 6 minutes, until the vegetables start to soften. Add the reserved orange juice mixture, and reduce the heat to low. Cook 1 to 2 minutes more, until the sauce thickens. Transfer the reserved chicken to a serving plate, top with the vegetables and sauce, and sprinkle with the flaxseeds. Serve immediately.

Kapha

4 tea bags, such as Darjeeling
1 pod star anise
1 cinnamon stick
1 teaspoon black peppercorns
2 limes, with peel
4 boneless, skinless chicken breasts
1 tablespoon peanut butter or almond butter
4 cloves garlic, minced
2 teaspoons hot chili sauce, such as Sriracha

2 teaspoons sunflower seeds
2 teaspoons ground flaxseed
1 tablespoon sunflower oil
2 carrots, thinly sliced
1 red bell pepper, seeded and thinly sliced
1 red onion, cubed
2 cups snow peas, cut into thirds
4 cups baby spinach leaves

Bring 8 cups of water to a boil in a medium saucepan. Add the tea, anise, cinnamon, peppercorns, and a 2″-strip of lime peel. Cover, turn off the heat, and steep for 10 minutes. Squeeze and discard the tea bags. Return the tea to a slow boil. Add the chicken, and cook 5 minutes. Cover the pan, and remove it from the heat. Let it stand 30 minutes or until the chicken is cooked through. Remove the chicken from the pot, and let it cool to room temperature. Slice the chicken into long, thin pieces. Set aside.

Meanwhile, squeeze the juice from both limes into a small bowl. Add the peanut butter or almond butter, garlic, and chili sauce. Whisk until smooth. Heat a large dry skillet over medium heat. Add the sunflower seeds and flaxseeds. Cook 2 to 3 minutes, stirring constantly, until the seeds are fragrant and toasted. Transfer to a plate. Heat the oil in the skillet over medium-high heat. Add the carrots, bell pepper, onion, and snow peas. Cook 5 to 6 minutes, until the vegetables start to soften. Add the spinach and the lime juice mixture, and reduce the heat to low. Cook 1 to 2 minutes more, until the sauce thickens and the spinach wilts. Arrange the reserved chicken on a serving plate, top with the vegetables and sauce, and sprinkle with the sunflower seeds and flaxseeds. Serve immediately.

PAD THAI

This dish will quickly become one of your favorites: It's a one-pot meal that is easy to pack for lunch, great to take on picnics, and dressy enough to serve to company. Fish sauce, rice noodles, buckwheat noodles, or soba noodles can be found in the Asian section of your grocery store.

Makes 4 servings

Vata

Pad Thai with Shrimp

    8 ounces wide rice noodles
    ⅓ cup lime juice
    ⅓ cup water
    3 tablespoons Asian fish sauce
    1 tablespoon rice vinegar
    2 tablespoons raw sugar
    2 teaspoons sweet chili sauce
    1 tablespoon canola oil
    2 cloves garlic, minced
    1 shallot, minced
    ½ pound shrimp, peeled, deveined, and cut into small pieces
    2 eggs, lightly beaten
    ¼ cup roasted, unsalted almonds, coarsely chopped
    2 cups bean sprouts
    4 scallions, thinly sliced
    ½ cup packed cilantro leaves, chopped

In a large bowl, cover the noodles with boiling water. Soak 20 minutes or until soft but not mushy. Drain, and set aside. Whisk together the lime juice, water, fish sauce, vinegar, sugar, and chili sauce in a small bowl. Set aside.

Heat the oil in a large skillet over medium-high heat. Add the garlic, shallot, and shrimp. Cook about 3 to 4 minutes. Add eggs, stir, and cook until still slightly moist.

Add the drained noodles, the reserved fish sauce mixture, the almonds, sprouts, and scallions to the skillet. Using a pair of tongs or 2 large spoons, toss until the noodles are evenly coated. Add the cilantro. Cook, tossing constantly, until the noodles are tender and the sauce has thickened slightly, about 3 to 4 minutes more. Serve immediately.

Pitta

Pad Thai with Tofu

    1 package extra-firm tofu (14 ounces)
    8 ounces wide rice noodles
    ⅓ cup lime juice
    ⅓ cup water
    3 tablespoons Asian fish sauce
    1 tablespoon rice vinegar
    2 tablespoons raw sugar
    ⅛ teaspoon cayenne
    2 teaspoons tomato paste
    1 tablespoon canola oil
    2 cloves garlic, minced
    1 shallot, minced
    2 eggs, lightly beaten
    ¼ cup roasted, unsalted almonds, coarsely chopped
    2 cups bean sprouts
    4 scallions, thinly sliced
    ½ cup packed cilantro leaves, chopped

Place the tofu in a colander and place a heavy pot on top of it to drain for 30 minutes. When the tofu has given off most of its liquid, cube it, and set it aside.

In a large bowl, cover the noodles with boiling water. Soak 20 minutes or until soft but not mushy. Drain, and set aside. Whisk together the lime juice, water, fish sauce, vinegar, sugar, cayenne, and tomato paste in a small bowl. Set aside.

Heat the oil in a large skillet over medium-high heat. Add the garlic and shallot. Cook about 3 to 4 minutes. Add eggs, stir, and cook until still slightly moist.

Add the drained noodles, tofu, the reserved fish sauce mixture, almonds, sprouts, and scallions to the skillet. Using a pair of tongs or 2 large spoons, toss until the noodles are evenly coated. Add the cilantro. Cook, tossing constantly, until the noodles are tender and the sauce has thickened slightly, about 3 to 4 minutes more. Serve immediately.

Kapha

Pad Thai with Chicken and Soba Noodles

- 7 ounces soba noodles
- 1/3 cup lime juice
- 1/3 cup water
- 3 tablespoons Asian fish sauce
- 1 tablespoon rice vinegar
- 2 tablespoons raw sugar
- 2 teaspoons sweet chili sauce, such as Taste of Thai
- 1 tablespoon corn oil
- 2 cloves garlic, minced
- 1 shallot, minced
- 2 boneless, skinless chicken breasts, cubed
- 1/4 cup roasted, unsalted almonds, coarsely chopped
- 2 cups bean sprouts
- 4 scallions, thinly sliced
- 1/2 cup packed cilantro leaves, chopped

In a large bowl, cover noodles with boiling water. Soak 20 minutes or until soft but not mushy. Drain, and set aside. Whisk together the lime juice, water, fish sauce, vinegar, sugar, and chili sauce in a small bowl. Set aside.

Heat the oil in a large skillet over medium-high heat. Add the garlic, shallot, and chicken. Cook about 5 to 6 minutes, until chicken is cooked through.

Add the drained noodles, the reserved fish sauce mixture, the almonds, sprouts, and scallions to the skillet. Using a pair of tongs or 2 large spoons, toss until the noodles are evenly coated. Add the cilantro. Cook, tossing constantly, until the noodles are tender and the sauce has thickened slightly, about 3 to 4 minutes more. Serve immediately.

DESSERTS

Granita

Granita is nothing more than Italian ice, but here it becomes a healing dessert. Vata's granita features orange, which is sweet, sour, and heavy, making it a perfect vata-balancing food. Cherries in the pitta recipe are cooling and also give the body strength and energy. And for kapha, pepper and cinnamon are combined with strawberries for a robust balancing concoction.

Makes 4 servings

Vata

Orange-Papaya Granita

1 small papaya, peeled, seeded, and chopped
  Zest and juice of 1 large orange
1 (1") piece ginger, peeled and grated
2 tablespoons honey
½ cup water

Place all ingredients in a blender or food processor, and blend until smooth.

Freeze in an airtight container, stirring and crushing lumps with a fork every hour, until evenly frozen, about 3 hours.

To serve, scrape with a fork to lighten the texture, crushing any lumps. Will keep for up to one month in the freezer.

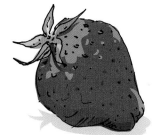

Pitta

Cherry-Basil Granita

- 2 cups frozen pitted black cherries
  Zest and juice of 1 small lemon
- 1 tablespoon (3 to 4 leaves) fresh basil
- 1 tablespoon (3 to 4 leaves) fresh mint
- 2 teaspoons raw sugar
- 1/2 cup water

Place the cherries, lemon zest and juice, basil, mint, and sugar in a blender or food processor, and blend until smooth. With the blender running, drizzle in the water.

Freeze in an airtight container, stirring and crushing lumps with a fork every hour, until evenly frozen, about 3 hours.

To serve, scrape with a fork to lighten the texture, crushing any lumps. Will keep for up to one month in the freezer.

Kapha

Strawberry-Spice Granita

- 2 pints strawberries, stemmed and quartered
  Juice of 1 lemon
- 2 tablespoons water
- 1 tablespoon honey
- 1/4 teaspoon freshly ground black pepper
- 1/2 teaspoon cinnamon

Place all ingredients in a blender or food processor, and blend until smooth.

Freeze in an airtight container, stirring and crushing lumps with a fork every hour, until evenly frozen, about 3 hours.

To serve, scrape with a fork to lighten the texture, crushing any lumps. Will keep for up to one month in the freezer.

Fruit Crisp

This classic American dessert is prepared with a twist—fresh herbs—but still has the crunchy topping that makes it so satisfying. The whole grain topping tastes just like the traditional version, but it contains ground flaxseeds, which are rich in omega-3 fatty acids.

Makes 4 servings

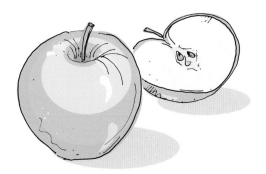

Berry Crisp

Filling

- 1 pint blueberries
- 1 pint strawberries, stemmed sliced
  Juice of 2 limes (about ¼ cup)
- 1 tablespoon fresh basil leaves
- 1 tablespoon whole wheat flour

Topping

- ½ cup rolled oats
- ¼ cup whole wheat flour
- 2 tablespoons ground flaxseeds
- ½ cup raw sugar
- 1 teaspoon baking powder
- ½ teaspoon cinnamon
- ¼ teaspoon salt
- ⅓ cup butter, chilled

Preheat the oven to 350°F. To make the filling: Place the blueberries, strawberries, lime juice, basil and flour in a small bowl. Stir well to coat the fruit with the flour. Transfer to an 8″ × 8″ baking dish.

Place the oats in a mini-chopper and pulse until a fine flour forms. Transfer the oats to the bowl of a food processor, and add the flour, flaxseeds, sugar, baking powder, cinnamon, and salt, and pulse 2 or 3 times to combine. Add the butter, and pulse 7 or 8 times, until pea-sized crumbs start to form. Do not overmix. Sprinkle the topping over the fruit, and bake 35 to 40 minutes, until the fruit is hot and the topping is cooked through. Cool 5 minutes before serving.

Apple Pear Crisp

Filling

2 apples, such as golden delicious or gala, seeded and thinly sliced

2 ripe pears, such as Bosc or Anjou, seeded and thinly sliced

¼ cup orange juice

1 tablespoon fresh mint leaves, chopped

1 tablespoon whole wheat flour

Topping

½ cup rolled oats

¼ cup whole wheat flour

2 tablespoons ground flaxseeds

½ cup raw sugar

1 teaspoon baking powder

½ teaspoon cinnamon

½ teaspoon cardamom

¼ teaspoon salt

⅓ cup butter, chilled

Preheat the oven to 350°F. To make the filling: Place the apples, pears, orange juice, mint, and flour in a small bowl. Stir well to coat the fruit with the flour. Transfer to an 8″ × 8″ baking dish.

Place the oats in a mini-chopper, and pulse until a fine flour forms. Transfer the oats to the bowl of a food processor, and add the flour, flaxseeds, sugar, baking powder, cinnamon, cardamom, and salt, and pulse 2 or 3 times to combine. Add the butter, and pulse 7 or 8 times, until pea-sized crumbs start to form. Do not overmix. Sprinkle the topping over the fruit, and bake 35 to 40 minutes, until the fruit is hot and the topping is cooked through. Cool 5 minutes before serving.

Raspberry Pear Crisp

Filling

1 pint raspberries

2 ripe pears, such as Bosc or Anjou, seeded and thinly sliced

Juice of one large lemon (about ¼ cup)

1 tablespoon fresh basil leaves

1 tablespoon whole wheat flour

Topping

½ cup rolled oats

¼ cup whole wheat flour

2 tablespoons ground flaxseeds

½ cup raw sugar

1 teaspoon baking powder

½ teaspoon cinnamon

¼ teaspoon nutmeg

¼ teaspoon cloves

¼ teaspoon salt

⅓ cup butter, chilled

Preheat the oven to 350°F. To make the filling: Place the raspberries, pears, lemon juice, basil, and flour in a small bowl. Stir well to coat the fruit with the flour. Transfer to an 8″ × 8″ baking dish.

Place the oats in a mini-chopper, and pulse until a fine flour forms. Transfer the oats to the bowl of a food processor, and add the flour, flaxseeds, sugar, baking powder, cinnamon, nutmeg, cloves, and salt, and pulse 2 or 3 times to combine. Add the butter, and pulse 7 or 8 times, until pea-sized crumbs start to form. Do not overmix. Sprinkle the topping over the fruit, and bake 35 to 40 minutes, until the fruit is hot and the topping is cooked through. Cool 5 minutes before serving.

Pudding Tartlettes

The rich and thick texture of these tartlettes resembles cheesecake, but they're made from low-fat protein sources (Greek yogurt for vata, and silken tofu for pitta and kapha) rather than heavy cream.

Makes 4 servings

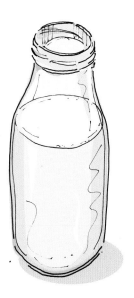

Vata

Crust

- ¼ cup white whole wheat flour
- ¼ cup rolled oats
- 3 tablespoons butter, chilled and cut into 1"-pieces
- 1 teaspoon raw sugar
- ¼ teaspoon salt
- 2 to 3 tablespoons ice water, or as needed

Pudding

- 3 eggs
- Juice of 4 limes + zest of 2 limes
- ½ cup fat-free plain Greek yogurt
- ½ cup maple syrup
- ¼ cup fat-free milk
- 1 tablespoon cornstarch

Preheat the oven to 350°F. Place the flour, oats, butter, sugar, and salt in a food processor. Pulse 4 or 5 times, until coarse, pebble-like crumbs form. Add the water, and pulse 2 or 3 times more until the crumbs are moistened. Press the crust into four 4″-round ramekins, and refrigerate.

In a large bowl, whisk the eggs, lime juice and zest, yogurt, maple syrup, milk, and cornstarch until smooth. Divide the mixture among the 4 ramekins. Transfer to a baking sheet, and bake 35 minutes, until the pudding is firm around the edges but still wiggles in the center. Cool completely on a wire rack. Cover, and chill at least 1 hour before serving.

Pitta

Crust

- ¼ cup all-purpose flour
- ¼ cup rolled oats
- 3 tablespoons butter, chilled and cut into 1"-pieces
- 1 teaspoon raw sugar
- ¼ teaspoon salt
- 2 to 3 tablespoons ice water, or as needed

Pudding

- 3 eggs
- ¾ cup silken tofu
- ½ cup reduced-fat coconut milk
- ½ cup raw sugar
- Zest of 2 limes
- 1 tablespoon cornstarch
- 1 teaspoon coconut extract

Preheat the oven to 350°F. Place the flour, oats, butter, sugar, and salt in a food processor. Pulse 4 or 5 times, until coarse, pebble-like crumbs form. Add the water, and pulse 2 or 3 times more, until the crumbs are moistened. Press the crust into four 4"-round ramekins, and refrigerate.

In a food processor, blend the eggs, tofu, coconut milk, sugar, lime zest, cornstarch, and coconut extract until smooth. Divide the mixture between the 4 ramekins. Transfer to a baking sheet, and bake 35 minutes, until the pudding is firm around the edges but still wiggles in the center. Cool completely on a wire rack. Cover, and chill at least 1 hour before serving.

Kapha

Crust

- ¼ cup all-purpose flour
- ¼ cup rolled oats
- 3 tablespoons butter, chilled and cut into 1"-pieces
- 1 teaspoon raw sugar
- ¼ teaspoon salt
- 2 to 3 tablespoons ice water, or as needed

Pudding

- ¾ cup silken tofu
- ½ cup maple syrup
- Juice of 4 lemons + zest of 2 lemons
- 1 whole egg
- 1 egg white
- 4 teaspoons cornstarch

Preheat the oven to 350°F. Place the flour, oats, butter, sugar, and salt in a food processor. Pulse 4 to 5 times, until coarse, pebble-like crumbs form. Add the water, and pulse 2 to 3 times more, until the crumbs are moistened. Press the crust into four 4"-round ramekins, and refrigerate.

In a food processor, blend the tofu, maple syrup, lemon juice and zest, egg, egg whites, and cornstarch until smooth. Divide the mixture among the 4 ramekins. Transfer to a baking sheet, and bake 35 minutes, until the pudding is firm around the edges but still wiggles in the center. Cool completely on a wire rack. Cover, and chill at least 1 hour before serving.

Grilled Fruit

Grilling fruit is one of the fastest ways to make a healthy and simple dessert. This version, made with fruits and spices appropriate for balancing your dosha— mangoes and cardamom for vata, peaches and cinnamon for pitta, and strawberries, pineapple, and cayenne for kapha—sets this sweet apart from others you've tasted.

Makes 4 servings

Vata

- ¼ cup balsamic vinegar
- 2 tablespoons raw sugar
- ½ teaspoon cardamom
- 2 large mangoes, peeled and thickly sliced
  Basil leaves for garnish

Place the vinegar, sugar, and cardamom in a small saucepan. Bring to a boil, and cook 4 to 5 minutes, until the liquid decreases by half. Coat a grill or grill pan with nonstick spray. Heat over high heat. Grill the mangoes 4 to 5 minutes, until the fruit has grill marks. Transfer to a platter. Drizzle with the balsamic sauce, and garnish with the basil leaves.

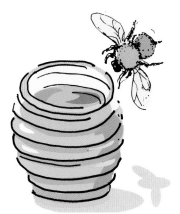

Pitta

   2 kiwi fruits, peeled
      Juice of 1 lime
   1 tablespoon honey
   4 yellow or white peaches, cut in half
      and pitted
  ½ teaspoon cinnamon
      Mint leaves for garnish

Place the kiwis, lime juice, and honey in a
food processor. Blend until smooth. Coat a
grill or grill pan with nonstick spray. Heat
over high heat. Grill the peaches 4 to 5
minutes per side, until grill marks appear and
the fruit softens. Transfer to a platter, and
drizzle with the kiwi sauce. Garnish with the
mint leaves.

Kapha

   5 strawberries, stemmed and sliced
   2 tablespoons water
   1 tablespoon raw sugar
   1 medium pineapple, peeled, cored, and
      cut into rings (1" thick)
  ½ teaspoon cayenne
      Mint leaves for garnish

Place the strawberries, water, and sugar in a
small saucepan. Bring to a boil, and cook 2 to
3 minutes, until the strawberries soften. Coat
a grill or grill pan with nonstick spray. Heat
over high heat. Grill the pineapple rings 4 to 5
minutes per side, until grill marks appear and
the fruit softens. Transfer to a platter, and
drizzle with the strawberry sauce. Garnish
with the mint leaves.

COOKIES

These cookies might taste like an old-fashioned recipe, but they are made with whole ingredients, such as oats and hazelnuts (vata), oats and coconut (pitta), and lemon zest and thyme (kapha).

Vata

Chocolate Chip Cookies with Oats and Hazelnuts

Makes 20 cookies (2 cookies per serving)

1/4 cup hazelnuts

1 cup rolled oats

1/2 cup + 2 tablespoons white whole wheat flour

2 tablespoons ground flaxseeds

1/2 teaspoon baking soda

1/4 teaspoon salt

1/2 stick unsalted butter, softened

1/2 cup raw sugar

2 egg whites

1 teaspoon vanilla extract

1/4 cup semisweet chocolate chips

Preheat the oven to 350°F. Spread the hazelnuts in a pie plate, and bake for 8 minutes, or until lightly toasted. Let cool, then coarsely chop.

In a small bowl, mix the oats, flour, flaxseeds, baking soda, and salt. Using an electric mixer, beat the butter with the sugar at medium speed, until light and fluffy, about 2 minutes. Add the egg whites and vanilla, and beat at medium speed, until blended, scraping down the side of the bowl as necessary. Beat in the flour mixture at low speed, until just incorporated. Using a large spatula, fold in the hazelnuts and chocolate chips.

Scoop heaping tablespoons of the dough onto 2 baking sheets lined with parchment paper, spacing them at least 1 1/2 inches apart. Bake the cookies for about 16 minutes, until lightly browned. Shift the pans from top to bottom and rotate from front to back halfway through for even baking. Let the cookies cool on the baking sheets for 5 minutes, then transfer them to a wire rack to cool completely.

Pitta

Chocolate Chip Cookies with Oats and Coconut

Makes 20 cookies (2 cookies per serving)

1 cup old-fashioned oats

1/2 cup + 2 tablespoons white whole wheat flour

2 tablespoons ground flaxseeds

1/2 teaspoon baking soda

1/4 teaspoon salt

1/2 stick unsalted butter, softened

1/2 cup raw sugar

2 egg whites

1 teaspoon vanilla extract

1/4 cups semisweet chocolate chips

1/4 cup unsweetened shredded coconut

Preheat oven to 350°F. In a small bowl, mix the oats with the flour, flaxseed, baking soda, and salt. Using an electric mixer, beat the butter with the sugar at medium speed, until light and fluffy, about 2 minutes. Add the egg whites and vanilla and beat at medium speed until blended, scraping down the side of the bowl as necessary. Beat in the oat mixture at low speed, until just incorporated. Using a large spatula, fold in the chocolate chips and coconut.

Scoop heaping tablespoons of the dough onto 2 baking sheets lined with parchment paper, spacing them at least 1$\frac{1}{2}$″ apart. Bake the cookies for about 16 minutes, until lightly browned. Shift the pans from top to bottom and rotate from front to back halfway through for even baking. Let the cookies cool on the baking sheets for 5 minutes, then transfer them to a wire rack to cool completely.

Kapha

Biscotti with Cranberries and Thyme and Lemon Glaze

Makes 16 biscotti (2 biscotti per serving)

- $\frac{1}{2}$ cup amaranth flour
- $\frac{1}{2}$ cup corn flour
- $\frac{1}{4}$ teaspoon baking soda
- $\frac{1}{8}$ teaspoon salt
- 2 egg whites
- $\frac{3}{4}$ cup raw sugar
- 2 tablespoons unsalted butter, softened
- 1 teaspoon vanilla extract
  Zest and juice of 2 small lemons
- 2 teaspoons fresh thyme leaves

Preheat the oven to 350°F. Coat 2 baking sheets with cooking spray. In a large bowl, whisk the amaranth flour, corn flour, baking soda, and salt. Using an electric mixer, beat in the egg whites at low speed until a crumbly dough forms.

In another bowl, beat $\frac{1}{2}$ cup of the sugar, the butter, vanilla, lemon zest (reserve the juice), and thyme, until combined. Scrape the mixture into the flour mixture, and beat at medium speed, until a soft, sticky dough forms.

Divide the dough into 2 mounds and transfer 2 to each baking sheet. Form each into an 8″-long cylinder. Pat the cylinders into loaves about 2″ wide and $\frac{3}{4}$″ thick. Bake for about 20 minutes, until the loaves are puffed and springy to the touch. Rotate the pans halfway through baking. Carefully transfer the loaves to a wire rack to cool for 10 minutes. Reduce the oven temperature to 200°F.

Using a sharp knife, cut the loaves crosswise into scant $\frac{1}{2}$″-thick slices. (Each will yield about 8 slices.) Return the slices to the baking sheets, each slice lying on its side, and bake for about 30 minutes longer, flipping after 15 minutes, until crisp. Transfer to racks to cool. Place the remaining $\frac{1}{4}$ cup sugar in a small saucepan with the lemon juice. Bring to a boil, and cook 1 to 2 minutes, stirring occasionally, until the mixture reduces by half. Cool slightly, then drizzle over the biscotti.

9

THE YOGA POSE INDEX
AND ILLUSTRATED GUIDE

We are like a field of wildflower swaying against the wind.
—Nikki Giovanni

This index is your home reference guide to keep you safe, healthy, and injury-free when you practice without a teacher to supervise your poses. Use the index in concert with the workouts that we prescribe for your type each week, or just browse through them and see what appeals to you.

We've encountered pose descriptions that read like a PhD thesis, so we wanted to streamline our how-tos. Each illustrated pose has very simple step-by-step directions.

When you approach yoga poses, the rule of thumb is to build your base first. Pay the most attention to your foundation by first planting your feet, then your legs. Then direct your hips, waist, torso, and shoulders. Then, when your body feels long and strong, incorporate your arms.

Follow the instructions until you have a good comfort level, and then begin to breathe deliberately. If you're more advanced and are ready to choreograph your breath and your movements simultaneously, match either the inhalation or the exhalation to each movement. If that feels too rushed, spend one full breath (inhale and exhale) in the position before you move on. You might want to stay in the pose for 3 to 5 more breaths before you move on.

One more piece of advice as you begin to peruse and play: Don't get caught up in self-talk such as "I'm not good at this." Take this advice when someone's poses (or this book's pretty illustrations) look more professional than yours: Everyone is searching for the same feeling, but it looks different on every body. If it feels good, you're doing it right.

Speaking of the illustrations, they are artful and elegant interpretations of the essence of each pose. If you are looking for exact anatomical depictions of poses, there are some great resources. YogaJournal.com is a fine place to start.

Your Yoga Pose Index

(continued)

Shoulder Stand

Side Plank

Side Plank with Single Toe Hold

Sphinx

Squat

Standing Split

Standing Yoga Mudras

Sun Salutation A

Sun Salutation B

Supported Fish

Tree

Tree with Lotus

Triangle

Twelve Point

Twisting Chair

Upward-Facing Dog

Warrior I

Warrior II

Warrior III

Windshield Wiper

Boat

1. Sit with your knees bent, feet flat on the floor. Grasp your legs under your thighs, slightly above your knees.

2. Lean back slightly. Lift your feet off the floor so your shins are parallel to the floor. Press the sides of your feet together.

3. Extend your arms straight out in front of you at shoulder height, with palms facing up.

4. Straighten and raise your legs toward the ceiling until your body forms a V shape.

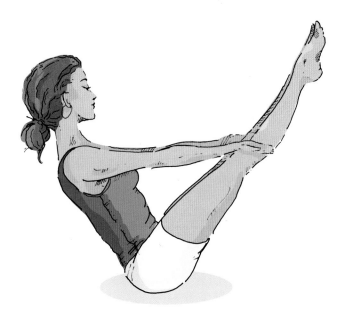

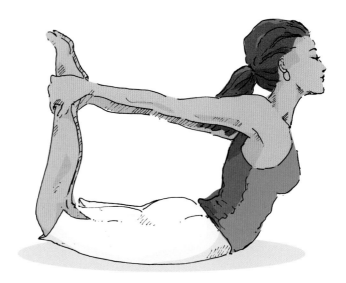

Bow

1. Begin in Sphinx.

2. Bend your right knee, bringing your right foot in toward your buttocks. Reach back to grab the outside of your right ankle with your right hand. Lift your knees off the floor.

3. Lower your right knee back to the floor, but keep holding on to your foot. At the same time, bend your left knee and reach back to grab the outside of your left ankle with your left hand.

4. Raise your chest and torso off the floor while simultaneously lifting your knees and thighs off the floor. Your hips and pelvis should be the only part of your body on the floor. Bring your gaze forward and slightly up.

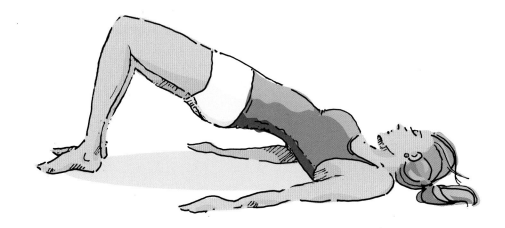

Bridge

1. Lie on your back with your knees bent and your feet flat on the floor. Keep your arms straight along the sides of your body, with your palms facing down. Your fingertips should touch your ankles.

2. Lift your hips and torso toward the ceiling. Make sure your knees don't splay out.

3. Interlace your hands beneath you and press your shoulders and upper arms into the floor as your hips lift higher toward the ceiling.

Bridge with Roll

1. Lie on your back with your knees bent and your feet flat on the floor.

2. Place a foam roller (or rolled-up yoga mat or towel) between your thighs. Squeeze thighs together to hold it in place. Place your hands by your heels.

3. Lift your hips and torso toward the ceiling. Keep your shoulders, hands, and upper back on the floor.

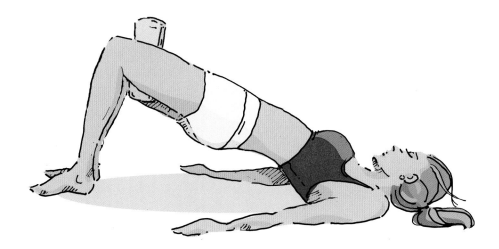

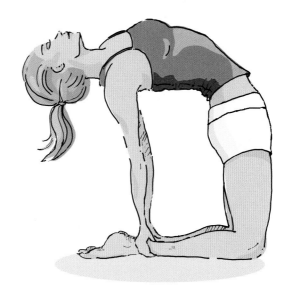

Camel

1. Kneel with your knees directly beneath your hips and your toes curled under or flat, depending on flexibility. Keep your shins hip-width apart and parallel to each other.

2. Place the palms of your hands on the small of your back, with fingertips facing up.

3. Lengthen through the sides of your body and lift your upper back up and over an imaginary ball.

4. Lower your right hand to your right heel or ankle and your left hand to your left heel or ankle.

5. Drop your head back gently.

Chair

1. Begin in Mountain.

2. Bend your knees, coming into a squat, but don't let your knees go forward beyond your ankles.

3. Straighten your arms overhead, with palms facing each other. Your chest should remain open.

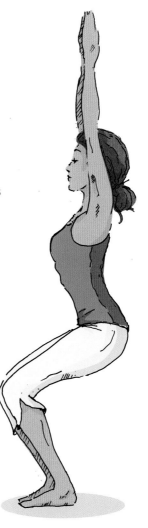

Child's Pose

1. Kneel on the floor with your knees about as wide as your hips.

2. Fold forward, resting your forehead on the mat and your torso against your thighs.

3. Rest your hands alongside your torso, palms up.

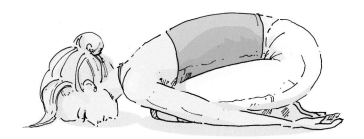

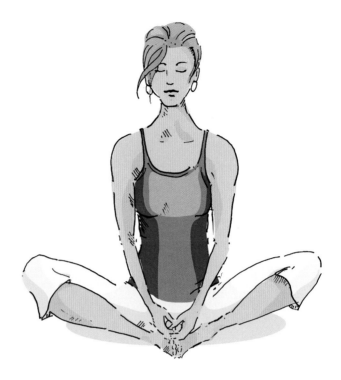

Cobbler

1. Sit on the floor with the soles of your feet together, holding your big toes with the first two fingers and thumbs of each hand. Lower your thighs toward the floor.

2. Keep your spine straight while slowly lowering your chest toward the floor.

Cobra

1. Lie belly down, toes and forehead pressing gently into the floor.

2. Place your palms next to your body along the sides of your chest, with your elbows bent and your fingers pointing straight ahead.

3. Press down into your palms, curling your shoulders and chest off the floor.

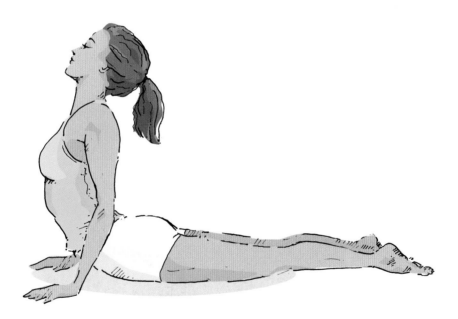

Corpse

1. Lie comfortably on your back on the floor. Move your arms about 1 to 1½ feet away from your body, with your palms up.

2. Extend your right leg to the right corner of the mat. Extend your left leg to the left corner of the mat. Relax.

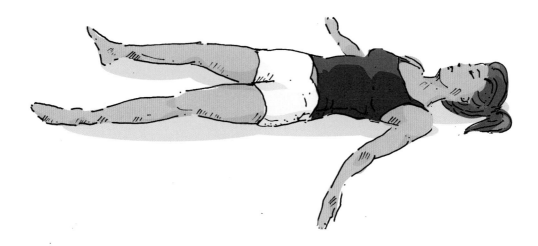

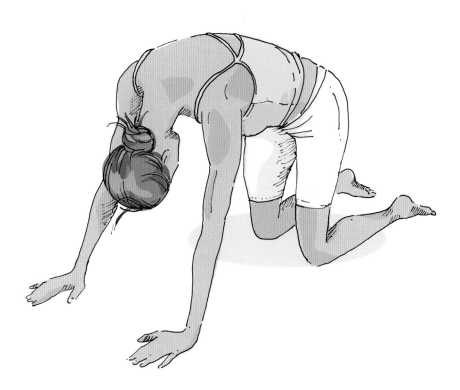

Cow/Cat

Cow:

1. Begin on your hands and knees. Curl your toes under.

2. Arch your back, lifting your chest, head, and tailbone up toward the
ceiling, pushing your belly toward the floor.

Cat:

1. While still on all fours, place the tops of your feet on the floor.

2. Round your lower back so that it reaches toward the ceiling while your
head extends toward the floor.

Cow/Cat Pointer

1. Begin on your hands and knees.

2. Raise your left arm in front of you, with your thumb pointing toward the ceiling.

3. Extend your right leg out behind you with the sole of your right foot facing the wall behind you and your toes pointing down.

4. Round your torso and bend your right knee, bringing your left elbow and right knee to meet under your torso.

5. Repeat on the opposite side.

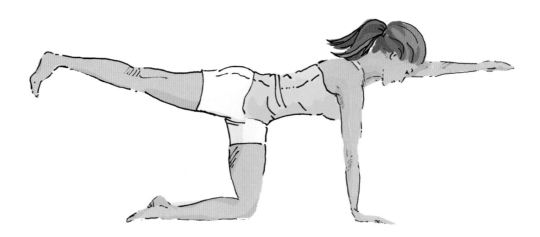

Cow Face

1. Sitting on the floor, bend your knees and cross your right leg over your left leg so your knees are stacked. Your right foot is just outside your left hip and your left foot is just outside your right hip.

2. Bend your right elbow up toward the ceiling, with your palm facing your back. Bend your left elbow to point to the floor, palm facing out. Reach your hands toward one another, grasping if possible.

3. Fold your body forward over your knees.

4. Repeat on the opposite side.

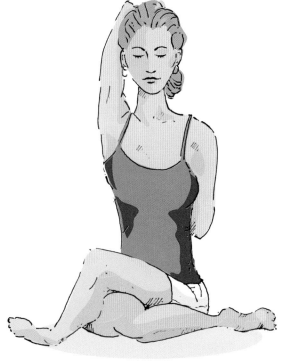

Crow

1. Begin in a Squat.

2. Place your hands flat on the floor in front of you so they are shoulder-width apart and your arms are bent.

3. Come on to your tiptoes, lift your hips toward the ceiling, and walk your feet closer to your hands.

4. Slowly shift your weight forward onto your hands and off your feet, until each knee is resting on each upper arm.

5. Transfer your weight fully onto your palms, causing your feet to float up behind you as your toes come together to touch.

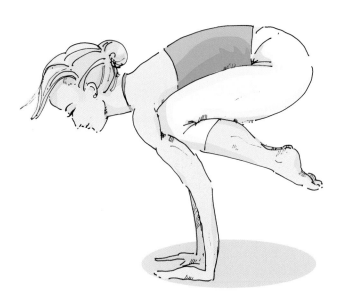

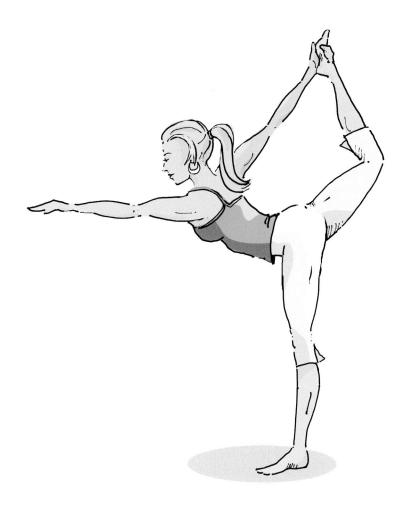

Dancer

1. Begin in Mountain.

2. Stand tall. Bend your right knee and reach back with your right hand to grasp your right foot. Your left arm extends forward.

3. Kick your right leg back. At the same time, lower your torso so your torso and your left arm are parallel to the floor.

4. Repeat on the opposite side.

Dolphin

1. Begin on your hands and knees.

2. Slide your hands forward until you are resting on your elbows and your arms are parallel, in a sphinx-like position.

3. Clasp your hands together so that your forearms create a triangle shape.

4. Tuck your toes under and straighten your legs, lifting your hips toward the ceiling.

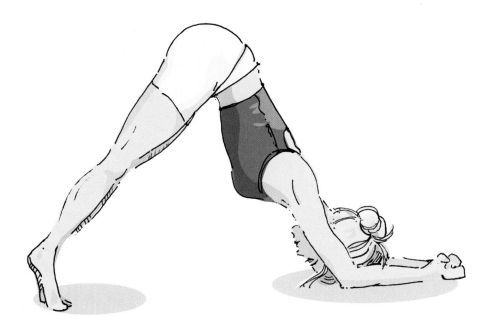

Double-Leg Forward Stretch

1. Begin in Seated Staff.

2. Lift your arms overhead, shoulder-width apart.

3. Keeping your spine straight, lower your chest and arms until your body forms a 45-degree angle.

4. Grasp your big toes with your first two fingers and thumbs.

5. Inhale, straighten your spine, then exhale, bend your elbows and lower your torso toward your legs.

6. When you cannot go any farther, lower your head toward your knees.

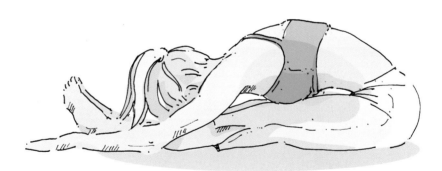

Double Pigeon

1. Begin in Cobbler.

2. Using your right hand, place your right shin on the floor, parallel to your body, with your right knee directly in front of your right hip.

3. Using your hands, place your left ankle on top of your right knee, then lower your left knee to rest on top of your right ankle.

4. Place your hands on your left leg.

5. Walk your hands straight out in front of you. Keeping your spine straight, fold your torso over your legs. Release your head to the floor.

6. Repeat on the opposite side.

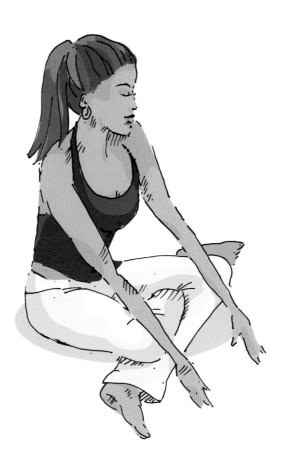

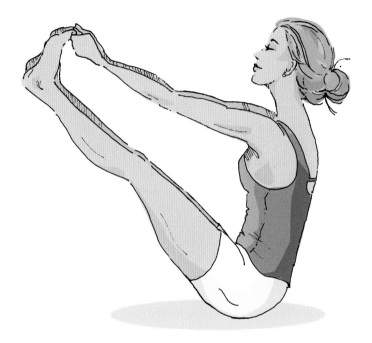

Double Toe Hold

1. Sit with your knees bent and your feet flat on the floor.

2. Grab each big toe with the first two fingers and thumbs of each hand on the same side.

3. Walk your heels in closer to your buttocks, and lean back slightly.

4. Lift your feet off the floor until your shins are parallel to the floor.

5. Continue lifting your shins until your legs are straight and your body forms a V shape.

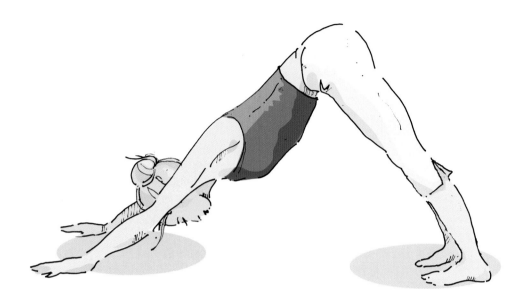

Downward-Facing Dog

1. Begin in Plank.

2. Lift your hips toward the ceiling so that your body makes an upside-down
   V shape with your feet flat on the floor, your hands turned slightly inward
   with fingers spread, and your arms extended.

Eagle

1. Begin in Mountain.

2. Raise your arms out to the sides to shoulder height with your palms down.

3. Cross your left elbow over your right elbow in front of your chest.

4. Bend your elbows, bringing your palms together.

5. Lift your right foot off the floor until your right thigh is parallel to the floor.

6. Cross your right thigh over your left thigh.

7. Wrap the toes of your right foot behind your left calf.

8. Lower your hips and bend your left knee, squatting more deeply.

9. Lower your torso toward your right thigh.

10. Lower your elbows to touch your right knee.

11. Repeat on the opposite side.

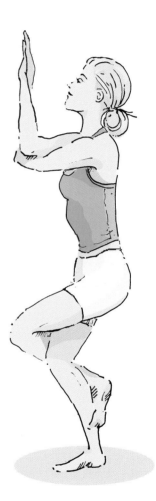

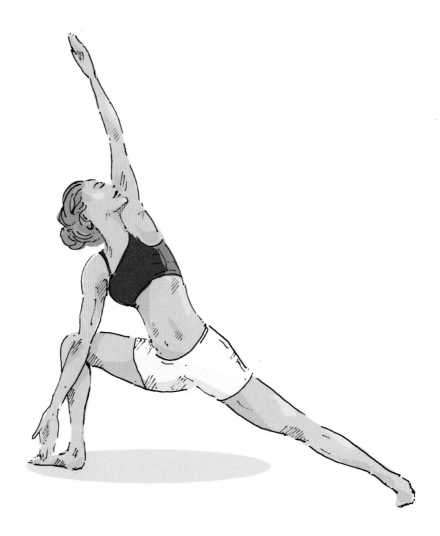

Extended Side Angle

1. Begin in Warrior II with your right leg forward.

2. Lower your right hand to the floor to the inside of your right foot. Place your left hand on your left hip.

3. Extend your left arm straight over your left ear with the palm facing the floor. Look up at your left fingertips.

4. Repeat on the opposite side.

Fish

1. Lie on your back with your legs straight in front of you and your arms along the sides of your body, palms down.

2. Press into your palms, and lift your chest toward the ceiling. Keep your forearms and elbows close to your torso and pressed firmly on the floor.

3. Lift your head slightly off the floor, then place the top of your head back on the floor.

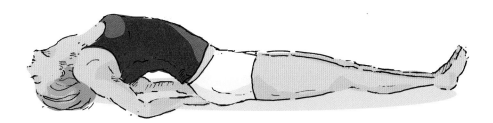

Flip the Dog

1. **Begin in** Downward-Facing Dog.

2. Extend your right leg to 90 degrees with your knee facing the floor.

3. As you open your hip, raise your leg high.

4. At your full extension, bend your knee.

5. Keeping your shoulders square, allow the big toe of your bent right leg to reach for your opposite shoulder.

6. Place the toes of your right leg on the floor, keeping the knee bent.

7. Move into a backbend, extending your right arm toward the front of the room.

8. Repeat on the opposite side.

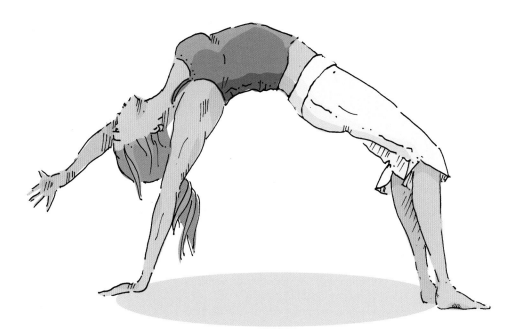

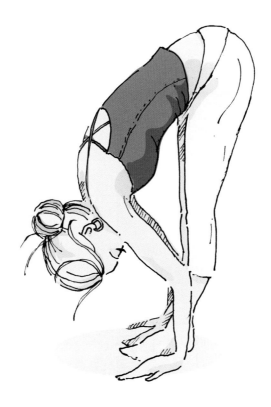

Forward Fold

1. Keeping your legs straight, fold your torso toward your thighs.

2. Rest your fingertips or palms on the floor. If you cannot reach, place your palms on your calves.

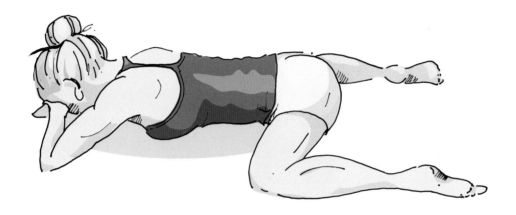

Frog

1. Begin on your hands and knees. Separate your knees as far apart from each other as you can. Separate your feet so they are the same distance apart as your knees.

2. Lean forward as you lower your torso to the floor.

3. Rest on your forearms.

Half-Moon

1. Begin in Triangle with your right leg forward.

2. Lower your left hand to your left hip. Slightly bend your right knee. Place your right fingertips on the floor about 12 inches in front of your right foot.

3. As you shift your weight onto your right leg, straighten your right knee and lift your left leg off the floor until it's in line with your left hip. The toes of your left foot face the wall to your left.

4. Extend your left arm toward the ceiling. Spread your fingers, and look up toward the ceiling.

5. Repeat on the opposite side

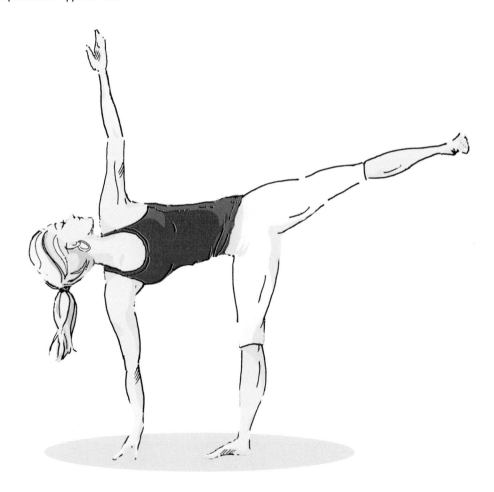

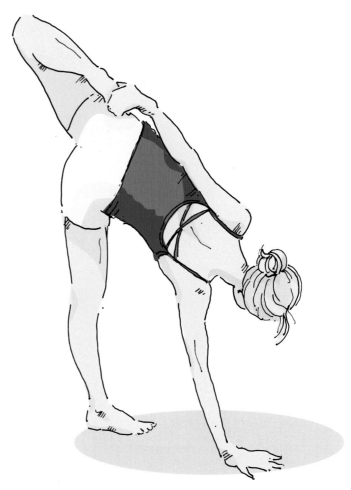

Half-Moon with Bent Knee

1. Begin in Half-Moon.

2. Grab your left big toe with your left "peace fingers" (pointer and middle finger).

3. Press your left foot away from your body.

4. Lift the foot skyward as you take a backbend into your upper back.

5. Repeat on the opposite side.

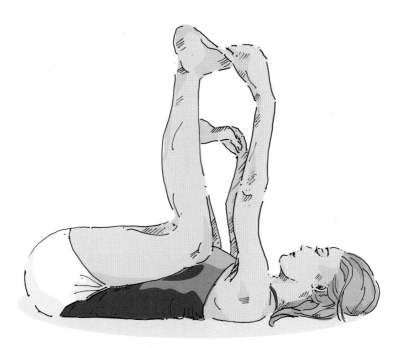

Happy Baby

1. Lie flat on your back. Lift both feet off the floor and bring your right knee toward your right shoulder and your left knee toward your left shoulder at the same time. The soles of your feet face the ceiling.

2. Grasp the outsides of your feet with each hand, pressing your lower back toward the floor.

Hero

1. Kneel with your ankles directly beneath your hips. Shins are hip-width apart and parallel to each other.

2. Lower your buttocks as you widen the distance between your feet and bring your knees closer together. The tops of your feet will be on the floor. Keep your thigh bones parallel, and sit up tall.

3. Slowly walk your hands behind you, resting your weight on your forearms. Gaze upward.

4. Release your back to the floor. Extend your arms along the sides of your body. Look up toward the ceiling.

King Pigeon

1. Begin in Pigeon with your right leg forward.

2. Bend your left knee so that your shin comes off the floor and your foot points toward the ceiling.

3. Turn your left palm toward the ceiling. Grasp the toes of your left foot with your left fingertips.

4. Rotate your left elbow out and up toward the ceiling.

5. Bring your left toes toward the back of your head as you bend back toward your foot, turning your gaze to the ceiling.

6. Repeat on the opposite side.

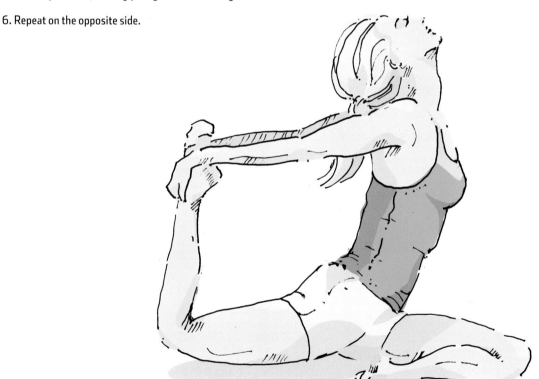

Kneeling Lunge

1. From Downward-Facing Dog, step your right foot forward between your hands, aligning your knee over your heel.

2. Lower your left knee to the floor.

3. Raise your torso and lift your arms overhead, drawing your shoulder blades down your back.

4. Repeat on the opposite side.

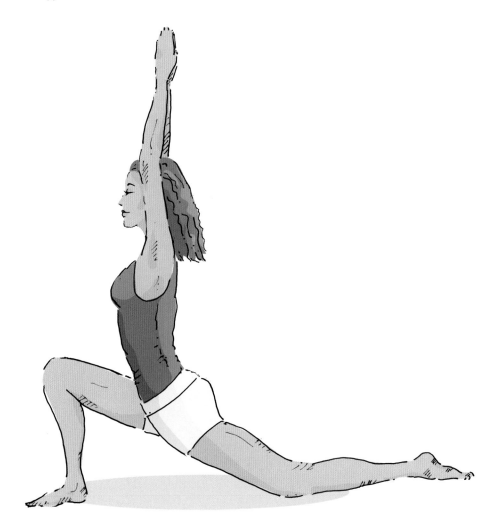

Legs Up the Wall

1. Sit with your knees bent and the left side of your body against a wall. Place your palms next to each hip.

2. Turn your hips to the left, and swing your legs up the wall while lowering your torso and head until they are flat on the floor, perpendicular to the wall. Your legs should extend straight up and against the wall. Stretch out your arms to the left and right, palms up.

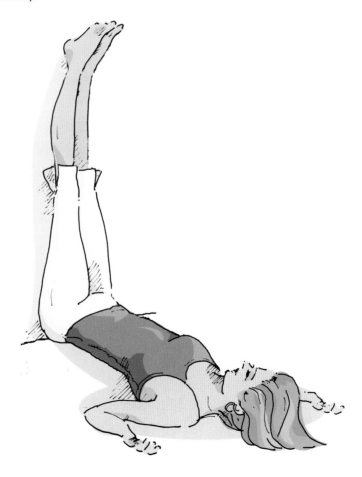

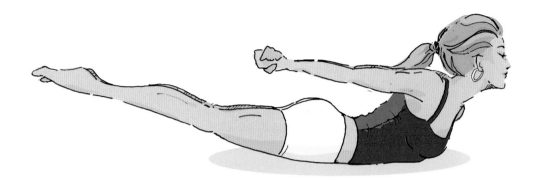

Locust

1. Lie belly down, arms along the sides of your body with palms facing up, your forehead and toes resting on the floor.

2. Interlace your fingers behind your back, and straighten your arms.

3. Keeping your arms straight, lift your chest, shoulders, and legs off the floor. Lift your arms several inches up, away from your body.

Lotus

1. From a cross-legged position, use the palms of your hands to draw your right ankle into the crevice of your left hip, with your foot facing skyward.

2. Place your left ankle into the crevice of your right hip, with your foot facing skyward. If your knees come up off the floor or your spine is compromised, sit on a pillow or block, or take only one ankle into the hip crease rather than both. (This is called a Half Lotus.)

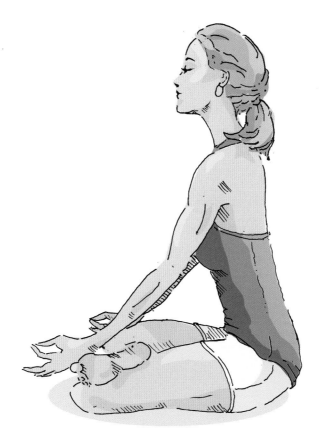

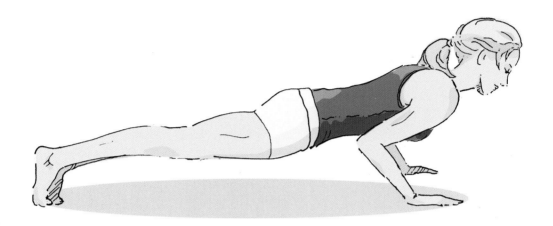

Low Pushup

1. Begin in Plank.

2. Bend your elbows and lower your body in a straight line toward the floor.

3. Hover about 2 inches above the floor with your elbows bent and pressing in toward your body, your upper arms in line with your torso.

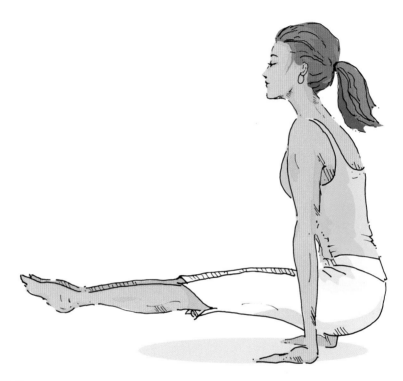

L-Seat

1. Begin in Seated Staff.

2. With your arms straight, press the palms of your hands into the floor and lift your hips and legs off the floor. The only parts of your body touching the floor should be your hands. If this is too much for you, keep your feet on the floor.

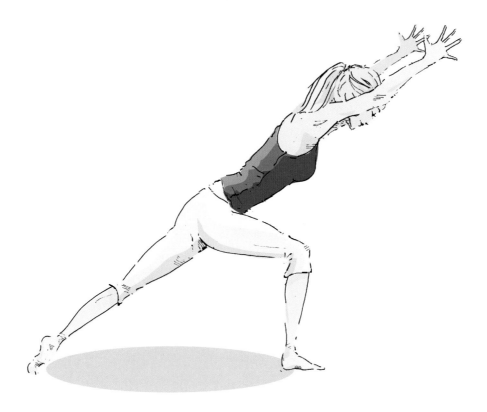

Lunge with Arms Power Forward

1. Begin in Warrior I. Rotate your back heel so that your toes face forward.
   Your front leg should remain bent, your knee aligned over your ankle.

2. Draw your shoulder blades down your back.

3. Extend your arms straight out in front of you, palms facing one another.

4. Lift your chest, extend your neck long, look at your mat.

5. Repeat on the opposite side.

Mountain

1. Stand with your big toes touching, heels slightly apart.

2. Lift your kneecaps and roll your thighs inward, tucking your tailbone underneath you and rolling your shoulder blades down your back. Let your arms hang at your sides, palms facing forward. You may raise your arms above your head.

3. Lift the crown of your head toward the ceiling.

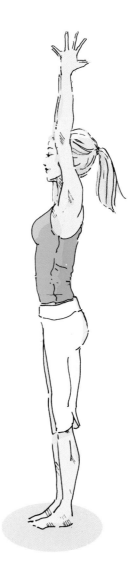

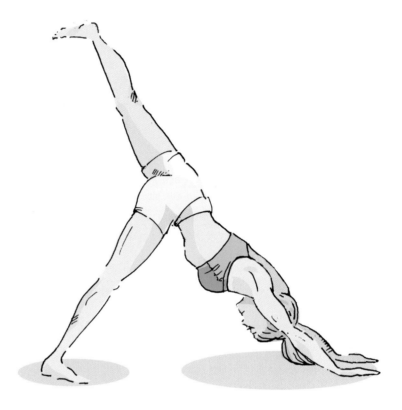

One-Legged Downward-Facing Dog

1. Begin in Downward-Facing Dog.

2. Extend your right leg behind you.

3. Keep your right knee facing the floor without raising or opening your right hip.

4. Repeat on the opposite side.

Pigeon

1. Begin in Downward-Facing Dog.

2. Bend your right knee in toward your chest. Turn your right knee out to the right, and place your knee on the floor with your right knee behind your right wrist and your right foot behind your left wrist.

3. Lower your hips, bring your left knee to the floor. Straighten your left leg, resting the top of your left foot on the floor.

4. Place your elbows on the floor with your forearms parallel to each other.

5. Stretch your arms straight in front of you, then fold your torso over your right leg, and lower your head to the floor.

6. Repeat on the opposite side.

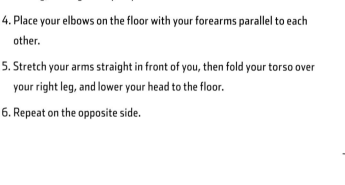

Plank

This resembles the "up" position of a pushup, with your arms extended and
your legs straight out behind you. Your body is in one straight, diagonal
line from your head to your heels.

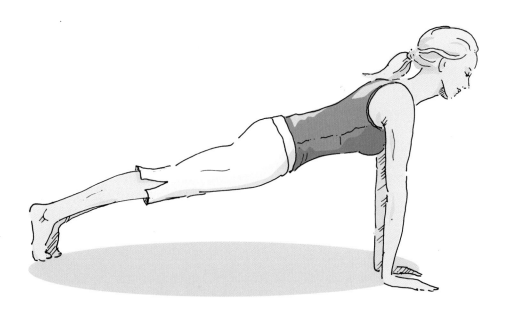

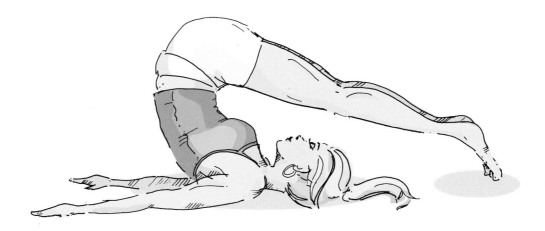

Plow

1. Lie on your back with your arms alongside your body. Bring your knees in toward your chest.

2. Extend your legs back over your head until the balls of your feet rest on the floor behind your head.

3. Clasp your hands behind you, and straighten your arms so that they are flat on the floor.

Prepare

1. Begin in Forward Fold.

2. Place your fingertips on the floor just outside your feet, with your fingertips in line with your toes.

3. Rise to your fingertips, straighten your arms, and lift your torso parallel to the floor.

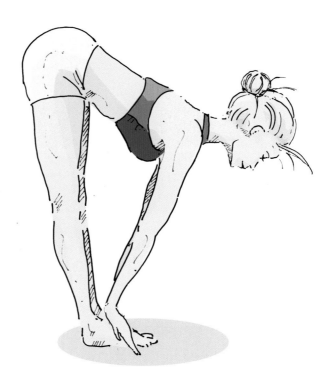

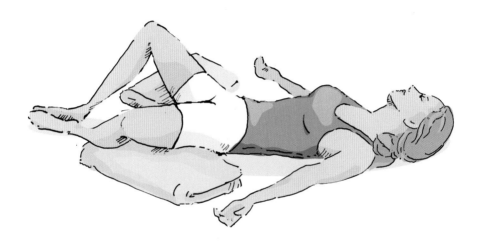

Reclined Cobbler

1. Lie on your back.

2. Bring the soles of your feet together into Cobbler.

Reclined Twist

1. Lie on your back. Cross your right thigh over your left thigh.

2. Let your knees roll to the left.

3. Bend your arms at the elbows with your forearms parallel to one another.

4. Repeat on the opposite side.

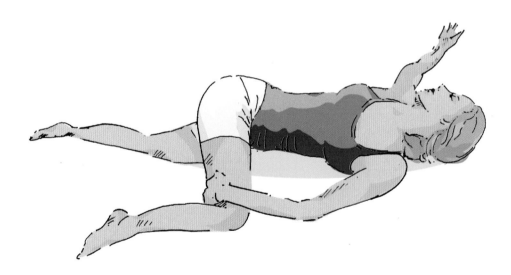

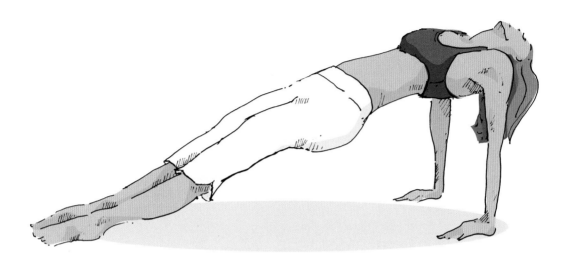

Reverse Plank

1. Begin in Seated Staff.

2. Press down into your hands. Lift your legs and hips off the floor.

3. Bring the soles of your feet toward the floor so your ankles, hips, and
   shoulders make a straight, diagonal line.

4. Allow your head to drop back slightly so your chin points toward
   the ceiling.

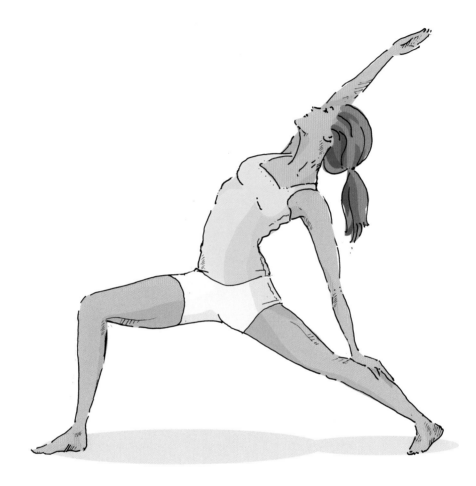

Reverse Warrior

1. Begin in Warrior II with your right leg forward.

2. Lower your left hand to your left calf (left fingertips pointing down).

3. Turn your right palm toward the ceiling, and arc your right arm up and
   overhead toward the wall behind you. Look up.

4. Repeat on the opposite side.

Revolved Half-Moon

1. Begin in Half-Moon, balancing on your right leg.

2. Rotating at the waist, place your left hand on the outside of your right foot.

3. Extend your right arm toward the ceiling, spiraling your chest toward the ceiling and looking up toward your right hand. Keep your hips level.

4. Repeat on the opposite side.

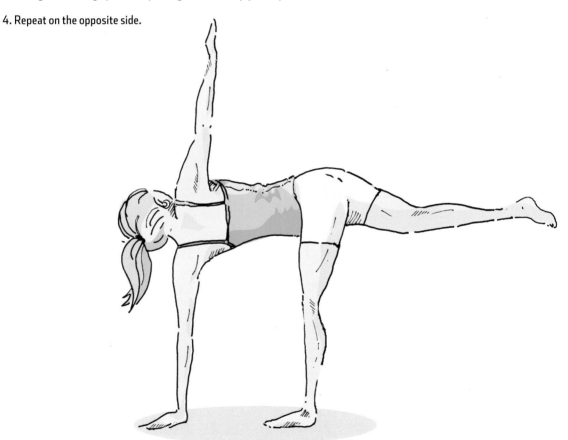

Revolved Triangle

1. Begin in Triangle Pose with your right leg forward.

2. Lower your left hand to the mat between your right foot and right hand. Press your left wrist against your right ankle.

3. Scoot your left leg in by 4 to 8 inches to shorten your stance.

4. Keeping your hips level and your back flat (parallel to the mat), raise your right arm toward the ceiling and look up at your right hand.

5. Repeat on the opposite side.

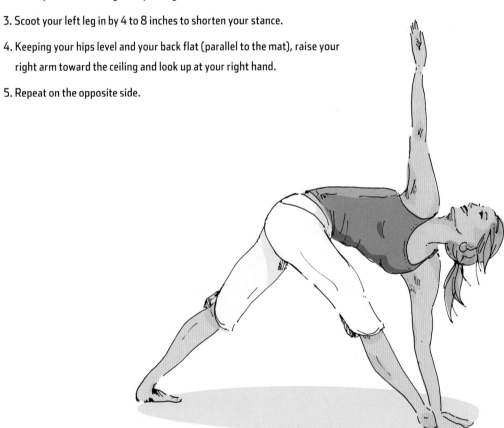

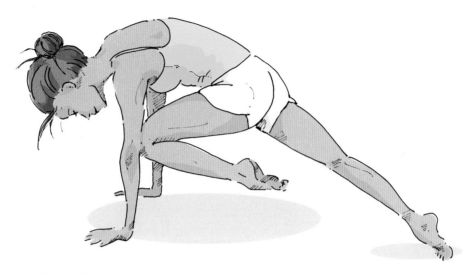

Rock 'n' Roll Pushup

1. Begin in Plank.

2. Draw your right knee up, bringing your kneecap toward your nose.

3. Draw your right thigh up toward the midline of your body.

4. Point the toes of your right foot, and squeeze your raised right leg into your body.

5. Repeat on the opposite side.

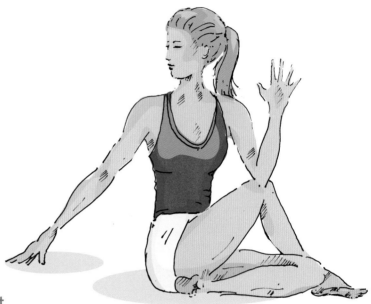

Seated Half Twist

1. Begin in Seated Staff.

2. Cross your right foot over your left leg, with the sole of your right foot on the floor on the outside of your left knee.

3. Bend your left leg so the heel of your left foot is next to your right hip. Lift your left arm toward the ceiling.

4. Bend your left elbow, and place it and your left upper arm on the right side of your right knee.

5. Place your right hand on the floor behind you, with fingertips pointing away from your body.

6. Press your left elbow and upper arm into your right knee, twisting your torso toward the wall behind you.

7. Repeat on the opposite side.

Seated Head to Knee

1. Begin in Seated Staff.

2. Bend your right knee and drop it to the right, then use your hands to bring your right heel closer to your groin.

3. Straighten your spine, place your left hand next to your left hip, and lift your right arm toward the ceiling.

4. Reach your right hand to the outside of your left ankle, then cross your left wrist over your right wrist.

5. Keeping your spine straight, fold your torso over your left leg.

6. Repeat on the opposite side.

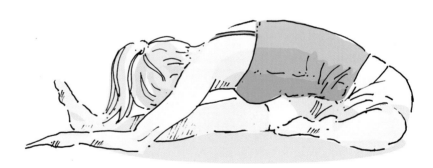

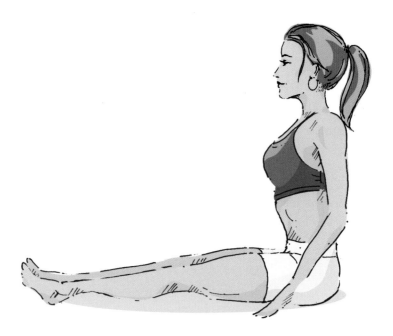

Seated Staff

1. Sit with your legs straight in front of you, with your toes pointing toward the ceiling.

2. Place your hands next to your hips, keeping your spine vertical. Look straight ahead.

Shoulder Stand

1. Lie on your back with your knees bent, your feet on the floor, hip-width apart. Your arms are by your sides.

2. Lift your feet off the floor, extending your legs toward the ceiling. Keep them straight.

3. Place your hands on your lower back, with your fingers pointing toward the ceiling. Gently pull your right and left arms closer to your body.

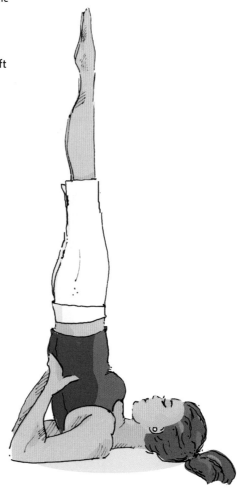

Side Plank

1. Begin in Plank.

2. Turn the toes of your right foot to face the left so the outside of your right foot is on the floor. Engaging your core, lift your left arm. Your shoulders should be stacked on top of one another so that your arms form a straight line.

3. Repeat on the opposite side.

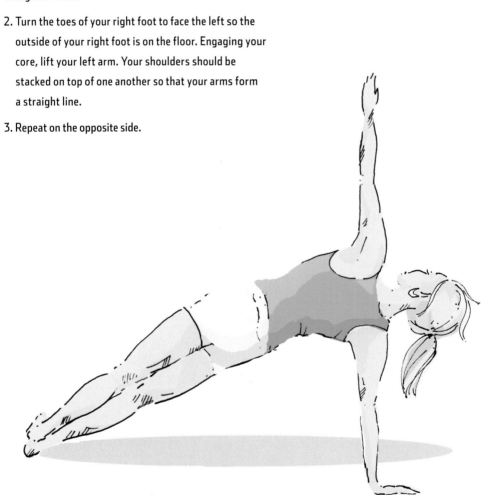

Side Plank with Single Toehold

1. Begin in Side Plank.

2. Draw the bottom of your left foot up your leg to the middle of your right inner thigh.

3. Hook your "peace fingers" (pointer and middle) around the big toe of your left leg.

4. Keeping your core and shoulder stable, extend the left leg, holding your toes until the extended leg and arm are straight and perpendicular to the floor.

5. Repeat on the opposite side.

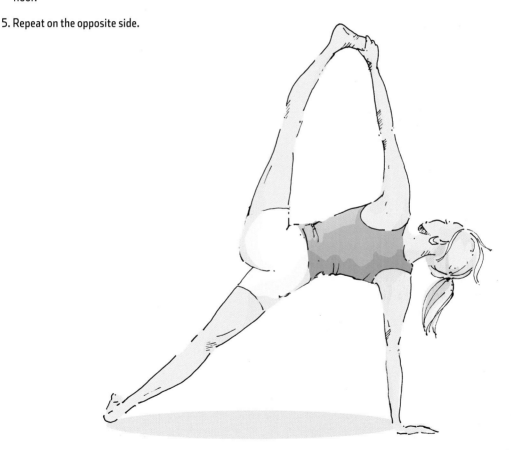

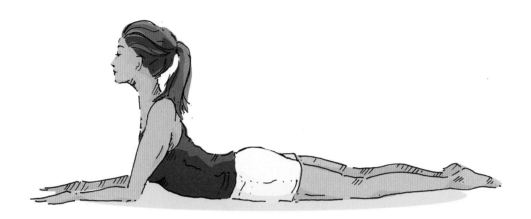

Sphinx

1. Lie belly down.

2. Place your elbows directly under your shoulders, your forearms on the floor in front of you, shoulder-width apart and parallel to each other.

3. Lift your chest off the floor, keeping your shoulder blades rolled down your back, and your neck long.

Squat

1. Stand with your feet slightly wider than your hips.

2. Bend your knees and lower your hips. Your heels should touch the floor. Your chest should remain open and your neck long.

3. Bring your palms together in prayer position at the center of your chest.

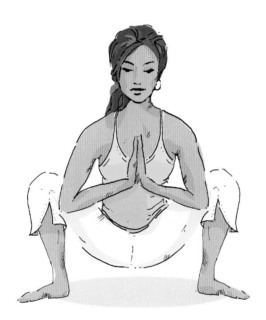

Standing Split

1. Begin Warrior II, with your right foot in front.

2. Twist to the right, lifting your left heel off the floor.

3. Lean forward, resting your torso on your right thigh.

4. Place your hands on the floor on either side of your right foot.

5. Shift your weight onto your right foot. Straighten your right leg,
   lifting your left leg behind you.

6. Repeat on the opposite side.

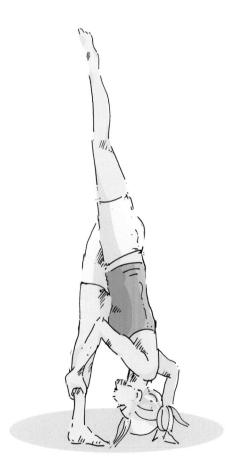

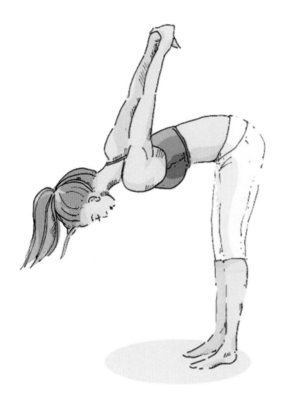

Standing Yoga Mudras

1. Begin in Mountain.

2. Interlace your hands behind your back. Straighten your arms, pulling your shoulder blades together. Look up toward the ceiling.

3. Fold forward from your hips, bringing your torso toward your thighs.

4. With your hands still interlaced and your arms straight, swing your arms away from your body as far as you can, aiming them toward the wall in front of you.

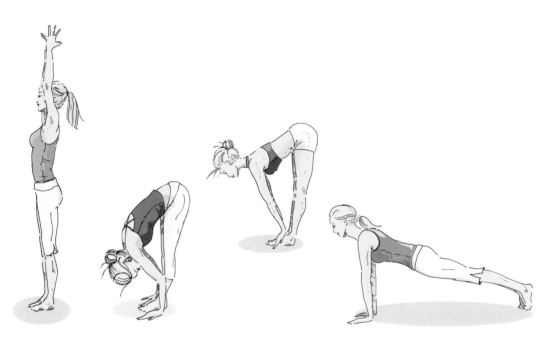

Sun Salutation A

1. Begin in Mountain.

2. Bring your hands together in front of your chest in prayer position.

3. Raise your arms toward the ceiling.

4. Forward Fold.

5. Keeping your palms on the floor, lift your torso until it is parallel to floor. Raise your head to look to the wall in front of you.

6. Jump back to Plank.

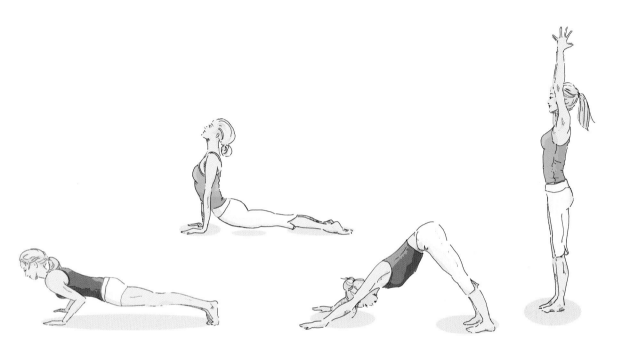

7. Low Pushup.

8. Upward-Facing Dog.

9. Downward-Facing
   Dog.

10. Step your right foot up
    between your hands.

11. Step your left foot
    next to your right foot,
    then straighten your
    legs coming into a
    Forward Fold.

13. Mountain.

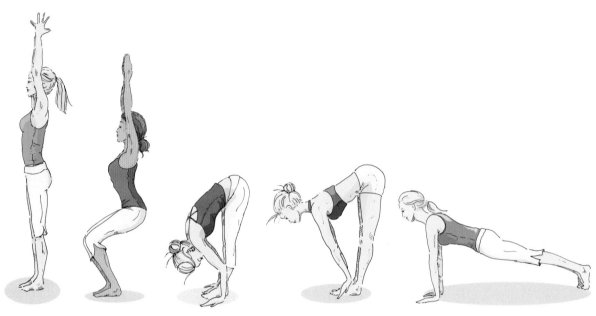

Sun Salutation B

Repeat sequence at least
twice, doing Warrior I on
both right and left sides.

1. Mountain. Raise arms
   above head.

2. Chair.

3. Forward Fold.

4. Prepare.

5. Plank.

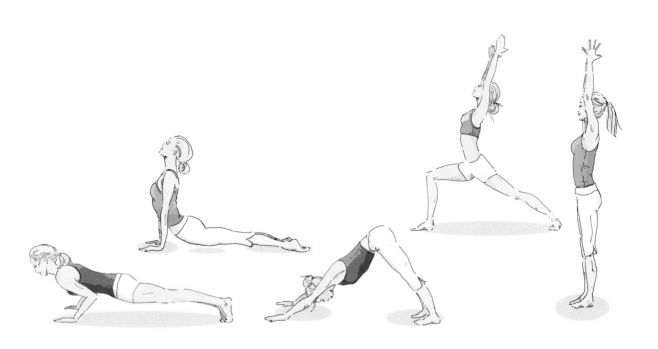

6. Low Pushup.

7. Upward-Facing Dog.

8. Downward-Facing
Dog.

9. Warrior I.

10. Mountain.

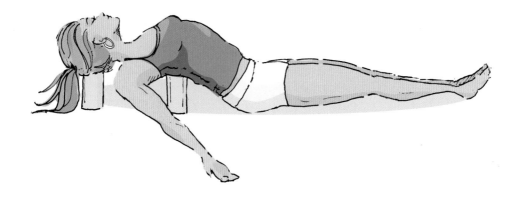

Supported Fish

1. Place two blocks on the floor about 18 inches apart.

2. Position one block beneath the nape of your neck and the other block in the middle of your back, beneath your shoulder blades.

3. Lie back over the blocks, with your legs straight.

4. Place your arms on the floor away from your body, palms up. Gaze upward.

Tree

1. Begin in Mountain.

2. Lift your right foot off the floor, turning your right knee out to the side. Place the sole of your right foot on the inside of your left leg, the heel of your right foot on your standing leg.

3. Bring your hands into prayer position in front of your heart.

4. Repeat on the opposite side.

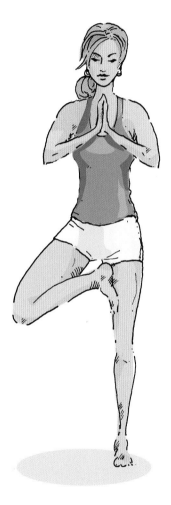

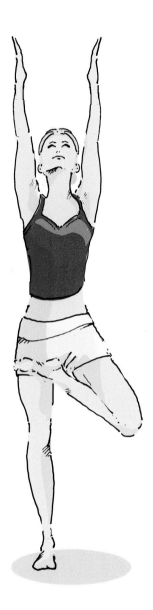

Tree with Lotus

1. Begin in Tree.

2. Using your hands, bring the outside of your right foot to the front of your left hip.

3. Bring your hands through prayer position and then lift them overhead.

4. Repeat on the opposite side.

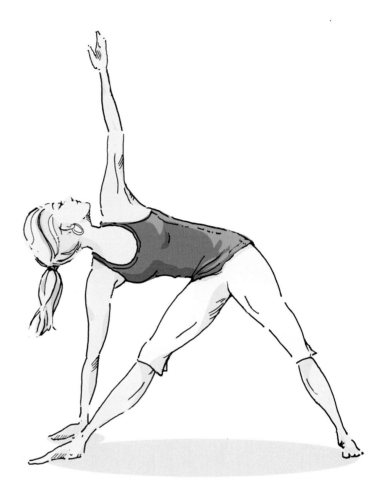

Triangle

1. Stand with your feet about 4 to 4½ feet apart, keeping them parallel. Turn your right foot and leg 90 degrees out to the right. Now turn your left foot in, toward the right, until it's at a 45-degree angle.

2. Raise your arms out to your sides at shoulder height, parallel to the floor.

3. Lower your right hand toward the floor, placing your right fingertips next to your right foot. Keep your legs straight.

4. Raise your left arm toward the ceiling, looking up at your left hand.

5. Repeat on the opposite side.

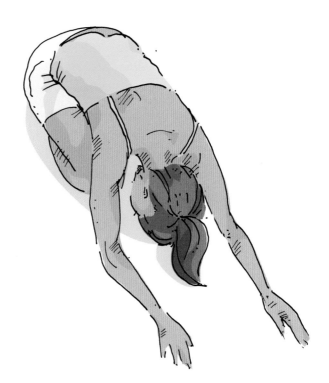

Twelve Point

1. Begin in Child.

2. Stretch your hands out in front of you, with your palms flat on the floor.
   Your right hand reaches toward the right corner of the mat while your left
   hand reaches toward the left corner of the mat.

Twisting Chair

1. Begin in Chair pose.

2. Bring your arms down, placing palms together in prayer at the center of your chest.

3. Twist your torso to the right and, swing your arms over to that side (hands still in prayer), placing your left elbow on the outside of your right knee.

4. Using your arms for leverage against your leg, turn your torso as much as you can. Your chest should remain open.

5. Look up at the ceiling.

6. Repeat on the opposite side.

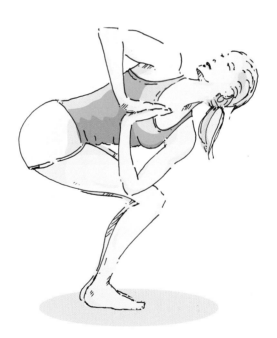

Upward-Facing Dog

1. Begin in Cobra.

2. Push down into your hands, straightening your arms and lifting your hips and thighs off the floor.

3. Arch your chest upward. Keep the tops of your feet firmly planted on the floor.

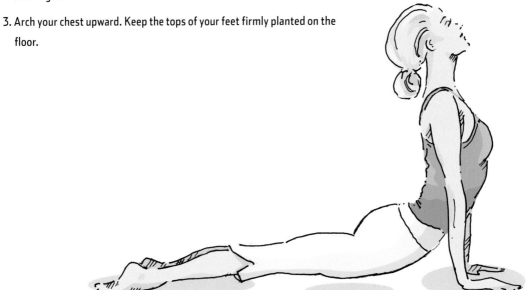

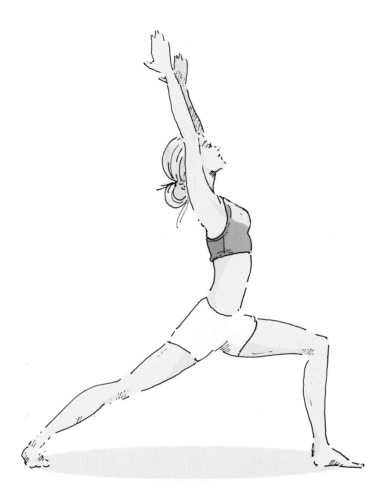

Warrior I

1. Stand with your feet about 4 to 4½ feet apart, keeping them parallel.

2. Turn your right foot and leg 90 degrees out to the right. Now turn your left foot in, toward the right, until it's at a 45-degree angle.

3. Rotate your hips and torso so they're facing the same direction as your right leg. Bend your right knee to form a right angle, your right thigh parallel to the floor. Lift your arms overhead with palms facing each other.

4. Repeat on the opposite side.

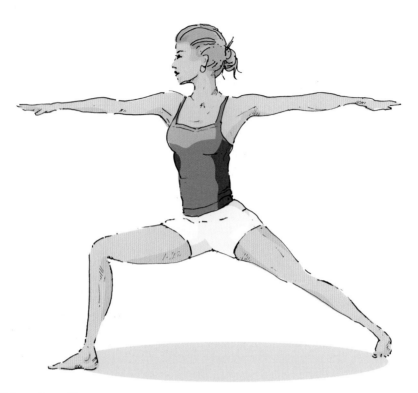

Warrior II

1. Stand with your feet about 4 to 4½ feet apart, keeping them parallel. Turn your right foot and leg 90 degrees out to the right. Now turn your left foot in, toward the right, until it's at a 45-degree angle.

2. Bend the right knee to form a right angle, your right thigh parallel to the floor.

3. Extend your arms out to the sides so they're parallel to the floor. Look over your right fingertips.

4. Repeat on the opposite side.

Warrior III

1. Begin in Warrior I with your right leg forward.

2. Bend at the waist and lean your chest down so that it's resting over your right thigh.

3. Shift your weight forward to your right leg. Straighten your right leg.

4. Lift your left leg off the floor and extend it straight out behind you. Your arms, torso, and left leg are parallel to the floor and both hips face the floor. The sole of your left foot faces the wall behind you, with the toes pointing down.

4. Repeat on the opposite side.

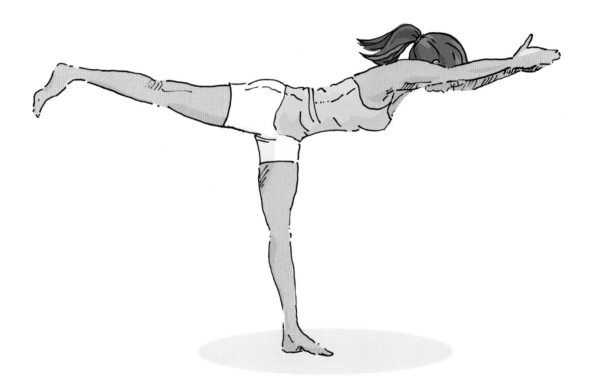

Windshield Wiper

1. Lie flat on your back with knees bent, feet flat on the floor. Arms are stretched out to the sides, palms facing up.

2. Shift hips slightly to the left.

3. Bring knees in to chest.

4. Keeping legs together, drop knees to the right.

5. Place right hand on top of left thigh; apply gentle pressure. Turn head to the left.

6. Repeat on the opposite side.

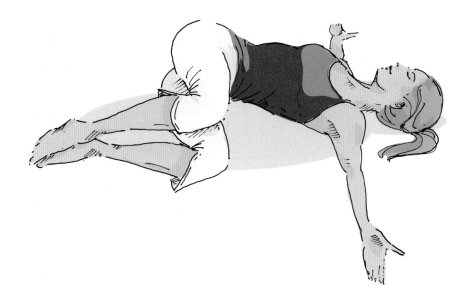

SAMPLE MENUS

Use the meal plans below, to put our recipes in Chapter 8 into action. For a list of Skinny Suppers, see pages 122–123.

WEEK 2

Day 1
Breakfast	Citrus Waffle
Lunch	Pesto Pasta
Dinner	Chopped Chicken Salad

Day 2
Breakfast	Breakfast Burrito
Lunch	Herbed Risotto
Dinner	Tasty Tacos

Day 3
Breakfast	Homemade Granola
Lunch	Fish in Phyllo
Dinner	Guacamole and "Chips"

Day 4
Breakfast	Fruit Carpaccio
Lunch	Tea-Poached Chicken with Vegetables
Dinner	Fried Rice

Day 5
Breakfast	Light-As-Air Crepes
Lunch	Superfood Sandwich with Creamy Vegetable Soup
Dinner	Rice and Beans

Day 6
Breakfast	Vegetable Omelet
Lunch	Dosha Burger with Salad
Dinner	Rice and Beans

Day 7
Breakfast	Berry Pancakes
Lunch	Tilapia for Your Type
Dinner	Vegetable Soufflé

WEEK 3

Day 1
Breakfast	Homemade Granola
Lunch	Pad Thai
Dinner	Skinny Supper of your choice

Day 2
Breakfast	Vegetable Omelet
Lunch	Roti Pizza
Dinner	Skinny Supper of your choice

Day 3
Breakfast	Light-As-Air Crepes
Lunch	Tasty Tacos
Dinner	Skinny Supper of your choice

Day 4
Breakfast	Fruit Carpaccio
Lunch	Herbed Risotto
Dinner	Skinny Supper of your choice

Day 5
Breakfast	Berry Pancakes
Lunch	Vegetable Soufflé
Dinner	Skinny Supper of your choice

Day 6
Breakfast	Breakfast Burrito
Lunch	Pesto Pasta
Dinner	Skinny Supper of your choice

Day 7
Breakfast	Citrus Waffles
Lunch	Fish in Phyllo
Dinner	Skinny Supper of your choice

WEEK 4

Day 1
Breakfast	Fruit Carpaccio
Lunch	Dosha Burger with Salad
Dinner	Skinny Supper of your choice

Day 2
Breakfast	Light-As-Air Crepes
Lunch	Chicken Quesadilla
Dinner	Skinny Supper of your choice

Day 3
Breakfast	Homemade Granola
Lunch	Tea-Poached Chicken with Vegetables
Dinner	Skinny Supper of your choice

Day 4
Breakfast	Berry Pancakes
Lunch	Roti Pizza
Dinner	Skinny Supper of your choice

Day 5
Breakfast	Breakfast Burrito
Lunch	Pesto Pasta
Dinner	Skinny Supper of your choice

Day 6
Breakfast	Vegetable Omelet
Lunch	Tilapia for Your Type
Dinner	Skinny Supper of your choice

Day 7
Breakfast	Citrus Waffle
Lunch	Herbed Risotto
Dinner	Skinny Supper of your choice

The Yoga Body Diet Online

www.theyogabodydiet.com

For more guidance and support, go to www.theyogabodydiet.com where you can find:

- Quiz yourself: Find Your Type.
- Download your FREE starter kit and workout plan.
- Yoga playlists for the workouts included in this book
- Cooking videos
- Yoga videos
- Shopping Sanity Savers

www.lifespa.com

Dr. Douillard publishes a bi-monthly video-newsletter on current health issues and the latest nutritional research. Currently he directs the *LifeSpa Retreat Center and Clinic* where he practices Ayurvedic and Chiropractic medicine in Boulder, Colorado. For more information or to sign up for his video-newsletter please find him at: www.LifeSpa.com or (866) 227-9843.

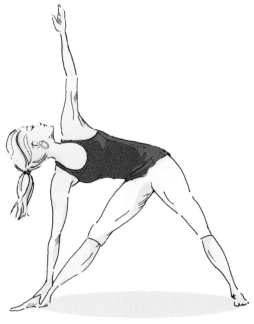

Index

Boldface page references indicate illustrations. <u>Underscored</u> references indicate boxed text.